AUSSIE BODY
DIET & DETOX PLAN

A happier, healthier you in just 14 days

SAIMAA MILLER

Photography by Rob Palmer

VIKING
an imprint of
PENGUIN BOOKS

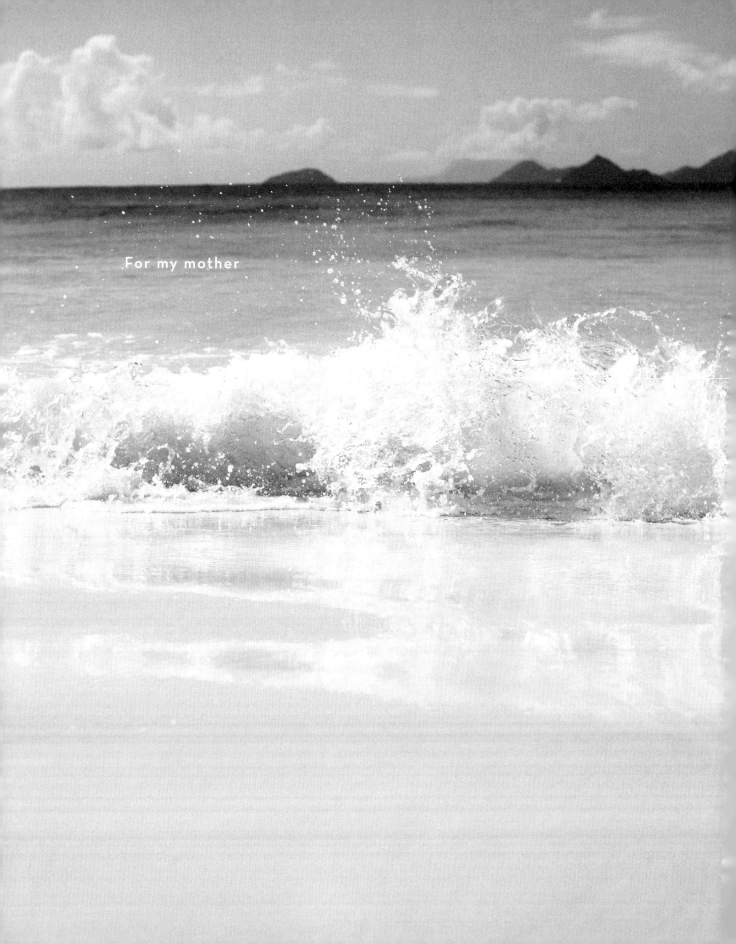

For my mother

CONTENTS

INTRODUCTION

Why do Australians look so amazingly healthy?
What's the secret?

Australia is not only a beautiful, diverse country; it's full of beautiful people. From the toned and bronzed specimens running along the beaches and yummy mummies pushing prams, to the Akubra-wearing guys mustering our cattle, Aussies are typically happy and healthy. Then there are our famous exports, such as Elle Macpherson, Hugh Jackman and Miranda Kerr. Australia has a well-earned rep for producing some of the sexiest and most vibrant people on the planet.

It's not dumb luck, nor is it coincidence. Aussies don't engage in restrictive diets or exercise excessively, count kilojoules, follow fads or gobble weight-loss pills. It's because a healthy lifestyle is synonymous with the 'Aussie Body'. Beautiful people fuel themselves with nourishing wholefoods; they make movement an integral part of their day; they get loads of sunshine; they think positively. We live a certain way which is why we look a certain way.

As a naturopath and detox specialist, I see Aussies from all walks of life: parents, celebrities, professionals, retirees, bohemians, and lucky for me, gorgeous elite sportsmen. What do they all have in common? They all want to look and feel their absolute best, and to live longer, side-step disease, have more energy, foster better relationships and eliminate stress.

But not everyone can go to a naturopath or visit a health spa. So I've created the Aussie Body Diet and Detox Plan, combining nutrition, detoxification, mindfulness and fitness, to show you – step by step – how to be truly healthy and exceptionally radiant, inside and out.

When you're firing on all cylinders, it shows. Bright eyes, shiny hair, clear skin, a flat stomach, oodles of energy and a mega-watt smile: all these things occur naturally when you're healthy. You can't get them with a magic pill. Being truly healthy means you're at your optimal weight without starving yourself. It means enjoying exercise because you can feel and see the results. It means feeding your body with the nutrients it craves. It means clearing out toxins. It means treating yourself with love and respect.

This book can change not only the way you look, but the way you feel. It is a road map to optimal wellness and will help you to reach your true potential in life. It's time to have these Aussie secrets revealed . . .

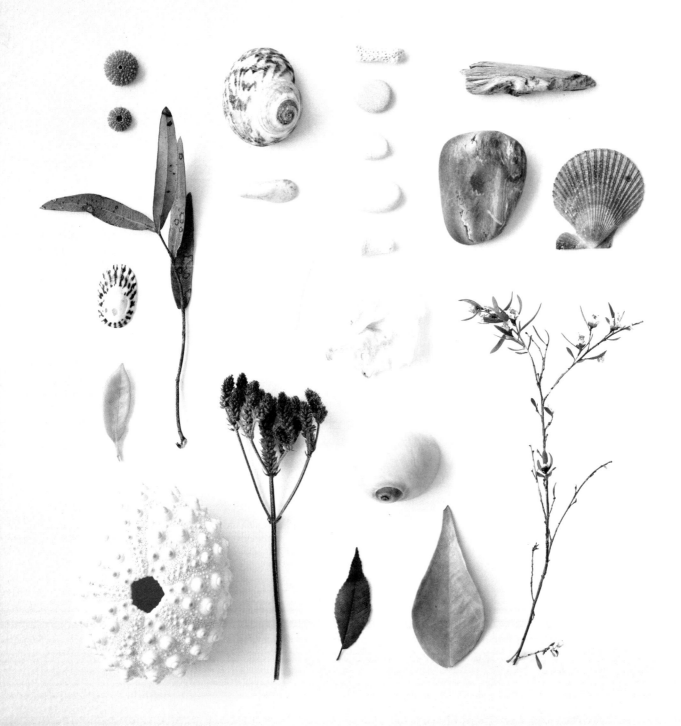

PART ONE

THE SEVEN AUSSIE BODY LIFESTYLE SECRETS

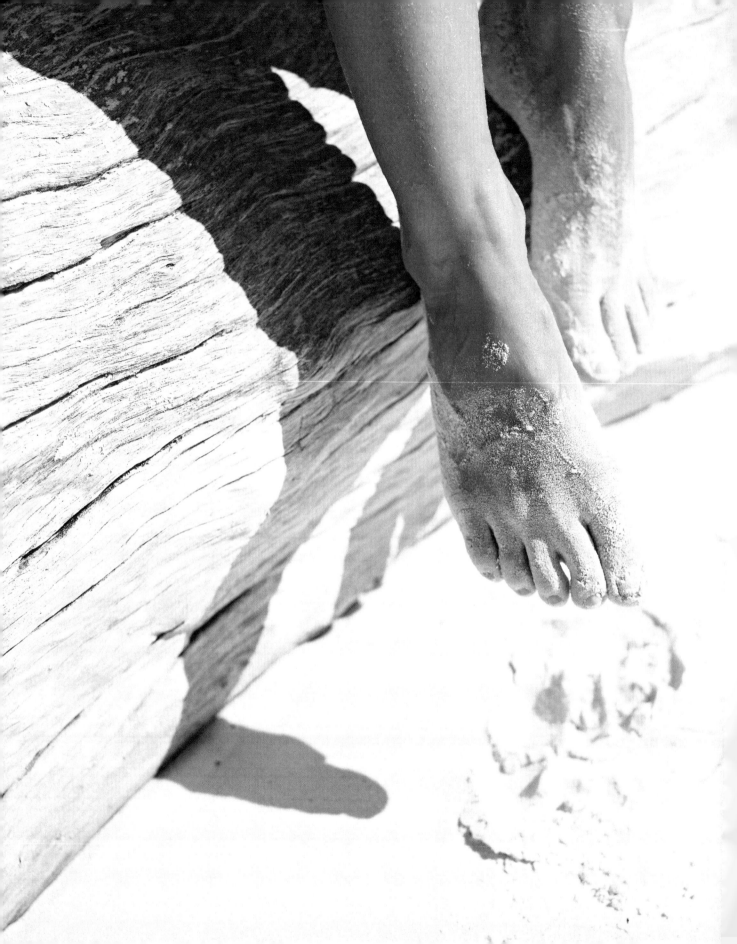

INTRODUCTION

Over the years, we've been bombarded with different ways to 'lose weight and feel great'. Watch your portion size! Don't eat carbs! Drink only lemon juice for a week! Eat grapefruit for breakfast! More recently, celebs have reportedly taken to the 500 diet: subsisting on 500 calories (2100 kilojoules) per day. Sounds about as healthy as an all-night drinking binge.

You'll be relieved to know that the principles described here are so much simpler. Most of my suggestions are based on common sense – what your intuition already tells you. It is what I call inherent knowledge, found in each and every one of us. These are the traditional principles passed down from our ancestors – lifestyle secrets for everyone to enjoy.

Part One is dedicated to these seven lifestyle secrets, which form the foundation of the Aussie Body Diet. You'll notice straight away that it doesn't comprise dogmatic formulas or restrictive rules – because true health and optimal wellbeing begins when you relax, let go of baggage, nourish your body and enjoy your precious life. When you allow yourself to be the best you can be.

Take advantage of these lifestyle secrets – they are written to guide you through the information overload we are now accustomed to receiving. The secrets have been around for centuries and the beauty in them is that they are so simple.

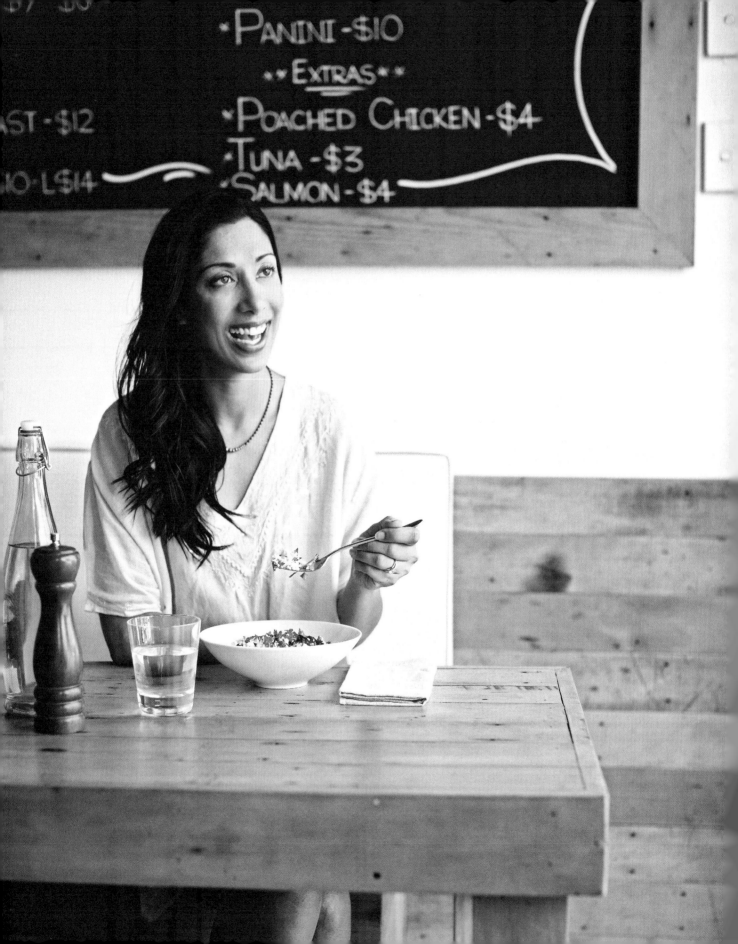

PANINI - $10
EXTRAS
POACHED CHICKEN - $4
TUNA - $3
SALMON - $4

AST - $12
IO · L $14

FOOD

'The gods are innocent concerning
the sufferings; all diseases
and pains of the body are the
products of extravagances.'

— Pythagorus, 500 B.C.

EAT LESS . . .

. . . and live longer. We don't need the amount of food that most of us in the Western world are accustomed to. The media and marketing industry has a lot to answer for: it often actively creates a 'need' to over-consume. Our ancestors were far more active than we are – and ate less food. Hands up who eats not only breakfast, but morning tea, lunch, afternoon tea, dinner and dessert? It's no wonder that the battle of the bulge has become an epidemic.

Often we think we're hungry right around the clock, because we're trained to over-consume. Food is abundant and cheap. Our stomachs are stretched. We crave food not always because we need to eat, but because we're *addicted*. Our body is an amazing piece of machinery; if you give it something regularly enough and in large quantities, it thinks it needs it. Cravings are a distress signal issued by the body when it's deprived of its addiction. But if you ignore the cravings, they'll go away eventually (I promise). And so will that extra layer of fat. You have to retrain your mind to let you eat what you need – no more, no less – and you achieve this by first transforming your eating habits.

Practise awareness. When you prepare your own food, you know exactly what you're eating. How many times have you baked a cake and been astonished at the amount of fat and sugar that goes into the mix? Touching, smelling and handling food before you eat it primes your body for digestion – think of Pavlov's dogs – and helps prevent overeating. Binging occurs when we skip meals and then over-compensate. Both overeating and binging can lead to obesity, which in

FOOD

turn places unneeded stress on the liver and digestive system.

Enjoy three meals spread evenly throughout the day, plus a snack or two if you're very active – or genuinely hungry. Allow yourself to feel hungry! It's your body signalling that it is time to eat, that you're not simply eating out of habit. When you're hungry, the wheels of digestion are already in motion. The enzymes in your saliva are champing at the bit, ready to break down much-needed sustenance. Bring it on.

Eat slowly. There's an old saying: 'Worry and hurry are the enemies of digestive health.' It's more relevant today than ever because we live in a fast-paced world where everything is instantaneous. You can download information in seconds on just about anything. You don't even need to leave your home to get food. Digestion begins in the mouth, where chewing physically breaks down food and the digestive enzyme amylase takes it from there. Eating quickly can lead to reflux, gas and bloating – because you're swallowing air as you gulp – and can provoke a condition known as 'leaky gut syndrome' where undigested food particles pass through the increasingly permeable gut wall, stimulating an immune response. This stimulates the immune system, which isn't ideal. It should be busy doing other things, like fighting bacteria and toxins. Many natural medicine experts believe that this increased gut permeability can cause everything from bacterial overgrowth to food allergies.

Savouring food and chewing well will also satisfy your tastebuds and allow your brain to get the message you're full, reducing overeating. So don't be embarrassed if you're last to finish at the table.

ENJOY WHOLE FOODS

Be cautious if a packaged food has a lot of ingredients. That means it's highly processed, and your body will have a hell of a time extracting nutrients from it – if there are any. Keep it simple. Fish is just fish, broccoli is just broccoli, nuts are just nuts, a banana is just a banana. You get my drift. Moreover, processed foods are often laden with more toxins, which are harmful in big doses. When you reduce your intake of toxins, your liver is freer for biochemical processes such as fat digestion. Your body runs at optimal capacity because it's not spending unnecessary time and effort mopping up toxins.

Genetically modified (GM) foods are also something to think about. GM foods were created out of a need to ensure an adequate food supply for our quickly multiplying population. There is evidence that the genes introduced into GM food attack what I call our 'bodily intelligence' and our internal environment. Over 70 per cent of processed foods have some type of genetically modified ingredient in them.

Eating whole, unprocessed foods is what our bodies need, love and truly crave. When you've got the time, prepare meals from scratch. Chop tomatoes yourself, peel and roast beetroot, roll your own sushi. Purchase a slow-cooker if you're time-poor and opt for healthy take-aways at dinner time if you're too tired to cook. Skip the sugar-heavy condiments and experiment with herbs and spices. Not all packaged food is highly processed, I know. But read the label – if anything has a lot of ingredients in it, you don't want it because it has been processed. Yep, this includes all those 'healthy' natural snacks too. And if the ingredients list boasts more numbers and unpronounceable words than a chemistry textbook, definitely don't eat it.

If possible, buy organic or 'clean' produce to limit chemical residues entering your body (and the earth). Certified organic food is free of residual synthetic fertilisers, herbicides and pesticides, and tastes so, so much better. You don't need to eat as much, because dense, nutrient-rich food offers abundant energy and fills you up.

If organic produce is hard to get where you live or it's just too expensive, purchase your food from growers' markets. At least that way you know the produce you are consuming is fresh, and a lot of growers' markets tend to stock produce that is free of chemical residues. It's good to know you're directly benefiting the farmers, too.

Eating organic or 'clean' fruit and veg helps you to be naturally aware of the seasons; it's important to eat foods that are appropriate for your body at different times of the year. It makes sense to enjoy sweeter, high-kilojoule fruits in summer, as we spend more time outdoors expending more energy. Winter is traditionally the time to eat root vegetables for their warmth and grounding qualities.

Animal and dairy products are often given a bad name but they are not 'bad' foods – no wholesome, unprocessed foods actually are. Opt for unprocessed animal and dairy products in moderation, making sure they form only a small part of your dietary intake, because these foods are quite acid-forming. Try to eat naturally raised meat – wild, free-range and organic are best – including fish, seafood, poultry, beef, lamb, game and offal (organs are particularly rich in minerals). Enjoy eggs, whole milk – not skim –and fresh cream and butter products from pasture-fed cows. I'm a big fan of fermented dairy, such as cultured yoghurt or kefir for their healthy gut flora effect (prebiotic and probiotic).

The key word here is 'enjoy'. Diets based on restrictive rules, portion control, and counting calories or kilojoules miss the point. Food is meant to be enjoyed. When you treat yourself to whole, unprocessed, nutritious foods, you don't need to worry about how many grams of fat or carbohydrates are in it. Forget about the glycaemic index. Forget about protein-only or grain-free. Stop labelling food as 'good' and 'bad'. Kick-start what I like to call your 'inherent bodily intelligence': your body knows what it wants and needs, and when enough is enough. Your body will show you symptoms of being unwell when you've eaten too much, or indulged in something that doesn't 'agree' with you. Lose the guilt and enjoy – and take the time to listen to your body.

A IS FOR ALKALISE

Alkalinity isn't just a buzzword seen on health blogs; many of us learnt about it in science at school. It's a familiar concept and I believe that achieving acid/alkaline balance in our bodies is imperative to long-term health and vitality. Our acid/alkaline balance is measured on the pH scale. The pH scale ranges from 0–14; anything below 7 (neutral) is acidic and above 7 is alkaline. Healthy blood has a pH of 7.4, which is slightly alkaline. Alkalinity is necessary for survival and our bodies have in-built mechanisms to ensure this acid–alkaline balance is maintained. If blood pH lowers (becomes more acidic), the lungs, kidneys and blood buffers naturally correct its level to a pH of 7.4. The human body is truly amazing.

So, what's this got to do with food? Well, I classify foods as acidic or alkaline, depending on how they affect the body after digestion. Just because a food *tastes* acidic, doesn't mean it is acid-producing. For example, lemons taste acidic but actually have an alkalising effect on the body after it's been digested (also known as alkaline ash).

Modern-day diets are a major contributor to acidity in the body.

The diets of our ancestors were much more alkalising than our diets are now. They were rich in fruits and vegetables, whereas today's diets contain more acid-producing animal produce, cereal grains and sugar – lots of it.

Unfortunately, many people today suffer from problems associated with too much acidity in the body. This over-acidic state can lead to health concerns such as weight gain, toxic build-up, fatigue, stress, lowered immunity, chronic pain and inflammation. In fact, natural medicine experts consider acidity to be the precursor to every illness ending with 'itis' (which is the medical term for inflammation).

I believe over-acidity is caused by dietary and lifestyle choices. It's exacerbated by processed foods and white-flour products, refined sugars, excessive red meat and dairy, crustaceans, alcohol, cigarettes, caffeine, soft drinks, food additives, preservatives and pharmaceutical drugs. Too much acidity in the body can also be caused by negative thinking and stress, even not stretching our bodies enough – more on all of this later.

An acidic environment inside our bodies is a breeding ground for pathogens such as candida albicans (yeast, commonly known as thrush) to live. Too much candida in our bodies is known to disrupt our digestion.

Moreover, our bodies only become addicted to substances in an acidic environment. When we choose more alkalising foods, our cravings for unhealthy foods, chemicals and substances actually disappear.

To help rebalance your body's pH, I advise you to avoid acid-producing foods and opt for alkalising foods (see Acid–Alkaline Chart on p 196). When your body is alkalised, you will feel energised, which means everything in your body functions as it's supposed to. You'll feel better, think more clearly and look healthier.

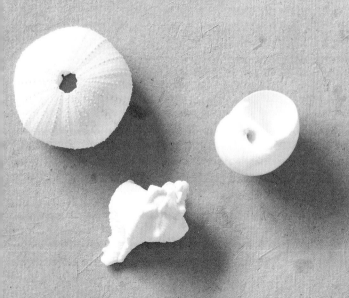

Choose alkaline foods full of chlorophyll. Chlorophyll (the substance in plants that make them green) helps supply vital oxygen to red blood cells. Chlorophyll is actually structurally similar to the haemoglobin in our red blood cells: we have iron in the centre of our haemoglobin, whereas the core of chlorophyll is made of magnesium – an important mineral for humans, too. (Research suggests that eating foods rich in magnesium can help prevent colon cancer.)

RAW FOOD ROCKS!

We're so removed from where our food comes from, and unfortunately love to cook it until it's unrecognisable. Many naturopaths believe that eating too many overcooked foods can contribute to chronic illness, weight problems and degenerative disease. Even the Big C. Acrylamide is a chemical that's been linked to cancer: it's the by-product of cooking foods, especially starchy carbohydrates, at very high temperatures. Significant levels of acrylamide are found in a wide range of packaged foods as a result of baking or frying. It can also be produced by grilling and roasting food to a certain degree. Eating charred barbeque meat is a big no-no. According to animal studies, the burnt bits contain heterocyclic amines, which can cause cancer.

Go for 50 per cent raw food, daily.
The less processed, the better. By heating or cooking food, we rapidly accelerate its 'death', as all health-giving nutrients in cooked food become degraded to varying degrees with cooking. I like to think of raw foods as 'live' foods. Imagine picking a perfectly ripe apple off the tree – it is still alive, with all its high-quality nutrients, water, fibre and cellular activity. Raw organic fruit and veg come to us straight from nature, not altered in any way. And because they take longer to munch and are oh-so-filling, raw fruit and veg will prevent cravings for fatty and sugary foods. Think about it: what takes longer to eat – a raw carrot or a Big Mac?

Enjoy raw foods: juice, fruit, uncooked vegies, sprouted grains and seeds, fermented foods and salads. You'll experience increased energy and vitality while boosting your metabolism, which allows your body to burn fat more efficiently.

GO GREEN JUICE: THE ELIXIR OF LIFE

Downing a Go Green Juice (see recipe on p 142) in the morning at least five times per week is the single most beneficial thing you can do for your body. It gives you a better kick than coffee and provides you with a boost of vitamins, minerals and electrolytes. If you make this a daily ritual, it will save you thousands of dollars in supplements and doctors' bills.

Choose dark, green, leafy vegetables such as kale, dandelion greens, silverbeet, spinach, beet greens, rocket, watercress, chicory, comfrey or mustard greens as your base. Then add vegies like beetroot, carrot, cabbage or celery. Throw in some alfalfa, coriander, parsley, mint, kelp, ginger or garlic for their detoxifying properties. Combine with low-fructose fruit to add sweetness while not disrupting blood sugar levels. Try apple (preferably green), kiwifruit or pear. Squeeze in alkalising fresh lime or lemon, as they're potent antioxidants. They also neutralise the bitter taste of green vegies. Hey presto, palatable juice! Finally, add oil, seeds and a superfood for extra rocket fuel – more on this later (see p 142).

You can use a blender to retain more of the fibre, but a slow-press juicer makes a nicer consistency that's easier to drink. Adding fibre in the form of seeds or meal is a great idea, too.

If you must have a coffee, always indulge after your Go Green Juice, never before. Having coffee on an empty stomach can muck up your blood sugar levels and stress your adrenal glands.

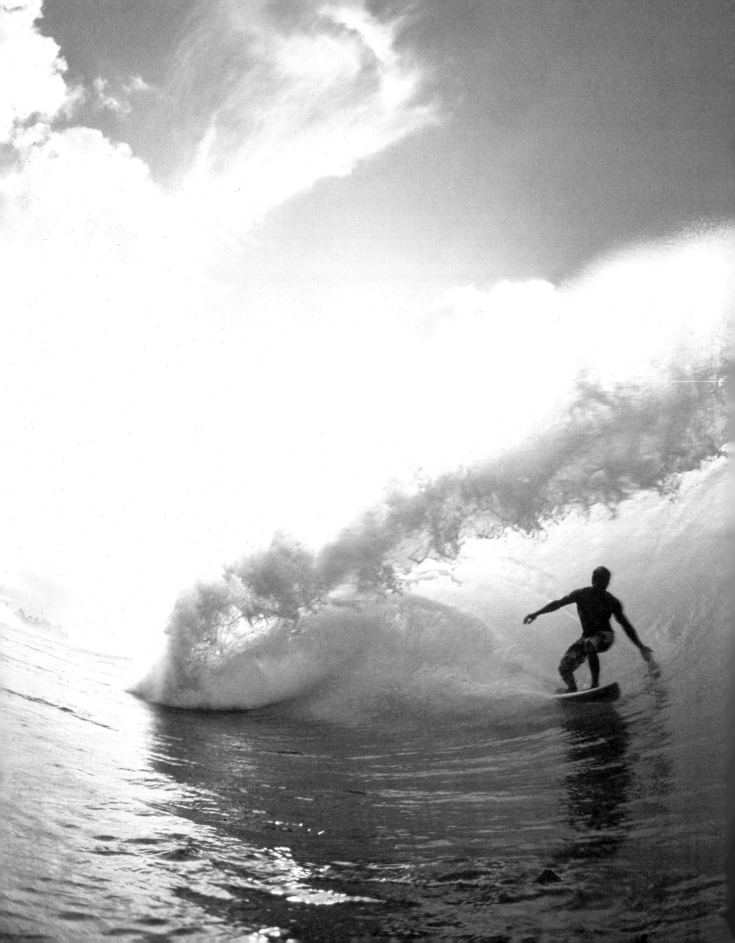

WATER

'When health is absent, wisdom cannot reveal
itself, art cannot manifest, strength cannot
be exerted, wealth becomes useless,
and reason is powerless.'

— Herophilus, 300 BC

WATER, WATER EVERYWHERE

Your body is made up of 75 per cent water and even a five per cent shift can negatively affect your health. The acid/alkaline balance determines your ability to hydrate: one study published in the *Journal of the International Society of Sports Nutrition* found the consumption of alkaline water – with a pH of 10 – improves hydration levels in young adults.

All of the cells of the body need water to stay healthy. After salt, water is one of the most important buffers of dietary and metabolic acid. If we don't get enough, our kidneys cannot filter wastes; when they don't work to capacity, some of their load is dumped on to the liver. One of the liver's primary functions is to metabolise stored fat into usable energy for the body. But if the liver has to do some of the kidneys' work, it cannot operate at full throttle. As a result it metabolises less fat, so more fat remains stored in the body.

Water is vital for the bloodstream to transport oxygen to cells, to regulate body temperature, and to maintain skin and muscle tone. Water is vital for your colon, or large intestine – one of the largest organs in the body. It constantly draws water from your waste material (aka poo) to be reused by the body, which is why you can be constipated when you're dehydrated. Water reduces the swelling in your brain when you're hungover. When we drink pure water we help our cells to transfer energy into our bodies – which basically means we feel more energetic! And the majority of nutrients dissolve in water, making water critical to being properly nourished. Without water, we can't absorb nutrients. We just can't live without water.

Water activates your metabolism.

Getting enough is possibly the single most important habit to form when you want to shed kilos. Researchers have discovered that water can boost metabolism by 30 per cent. Another trial found that drinking water before a meal leads to greater weight loss – because it fills you up before you can say 'chicken parmigiana'. (Just make sure you're not drinking your water directly before meals as natural medicine experts believe this will dilute your digestive enzymes).

Don't take water for granted; it may be the only true magic potion for permanent weight loss. Often you might think you're hungry when, in fact, you're simply dehydrated. Our bodies also have great difficulty metabolising stored body fat unless we drink sufficient amounts of water. If you were stuck in a desert without water, your body would slow down your metabolism as a survival mechanism. This means your body stores fat rather than using it. So if you drink less water, your body will store more fat, while if you drink more water, your body will burn the fat for energy.

The water also helps to flush out the metabolised fat that your body produces as waste when you are losing weight. So scull a glass of water to curb hunger pangs (when it's not time to eat, and you'll find the hunger will just go).

Drinking enough water is one of the best treatments for fluid retention (oedema), when the lymphatic system isn't draining water from the body's tissues effectively. People who suffer from oedema mistakenly believe drinking more water will exacerbate the condition. Wrong. Give your body plenty of water and seek advice from a health practitioner – oedema may be indicative of an underlying dysfunction. Best to get to the root of the problem.

You're not a camel. Drink up!

I can't say this enough: guzzling filtered water every day is the best way to nurture your body. And I'm talking about more than the recommended eight glasses. That equals two litres of water, but we lose an average of two and a half litres of water every day. Wow. At least three litres daily is necessary for optimal health. You need more if you're overweight, do lots of physical activity or spend time in heated or air-conditioned environments. In the summer time, drink some more.

If you're not a big drinker, don't jump straight to three litres a day. Take it slow. Start with 500 ml on rising, then 500 ml mid-morning, followed by mid-afternoon and after dinner. After a few days, increase it to 750 ml at the same times. Don't worry if you visit the bathroom more frequently – this settles. The bladder's sphincter is a muscle and like all muscles, it needs to be exercised. The urge to pee will become, well, less urgent. The most important thing to pay attention to with water is *when* you drink it – that is, drink your main bulk of water away from meals, and just sip water if needed at meal times.

Drinking water at room temperature is easy on the body, because our internal environment optimally runs at 37.5°C. Meanwhile, there's evidence to suggest that drinking cold water can burn more kilojoules, as your body's expending energy to warm the water to body temperature. I prefer room-temperature water, but don't sweat the small stuff. The important thing is you're drinking (lots of) water.

If you can, opt for spring water. Or natural mineral water. As the name suggests, it boasts the minerals magnesium and calcium, which are oh-so-good for you. Plain tap water isn't the best choice, sorry. Although it's treated and filtered, it can still contain contaminants such as pesticide residue, micro-organisms and heavy metals. Then there's added fluoride, the benefits of which are debatable. Some researchers believe fluoride may do more harm than good.

Go one better: drink alkaline water. I won't bore you with a chemistry lesson, but alkaline water goes through the process of ionisation. The water is separated into alkaline and acid streams, leaving just the alkaline water, made of 'micro-clusters' that cross cell walls faster. I'm a huge fan of alkaline water because it results in super-quick hydration and easy delivery of nutrients to cells, while neutralising acids in the body. Alkaline water is a powerful antioxidant.

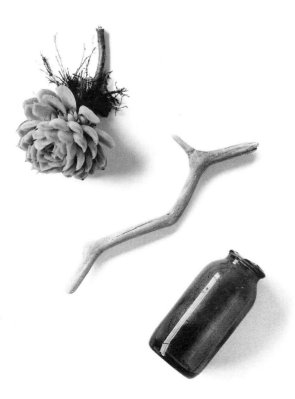

SEA SALT: GUILT-FREE FLAVOUR

We're constantly told that salt is bad for us. But unrefined sea salt – not table salt – can do wonders. Salt water in the form of a saline spray is used to treat asthma and cystic fibrosis. It can stop a persistent dry cough *and* clear mucus from lungs. Gargling salt water is an effective remedy for a sore throat. Bathing in salt water can alleviate eczema and psoriasis; the Dead Sea community have been doing it for thousands of years. Salt is a strong antiseptic.

When looking for sea salt to use in cooking, ensure it's been evaporated by the sun and not kiln-dried. Kiln-drying scorches the salt at a high temperature to remove moisture, which can deplete trace minerals such as calcium, magnesium and potassium. It's harder on the body. Even some 'natural sea salts' have been kiln-dried, so do your research.

Many brands of common table salt contain unnatural anti-caking agents. This 'bad' salt is added to a lot of processed food and takeaways. Eat too much convenience food and you'll easily clock up more than the recommended 4 g (1600 mg sodium) of salt per day.

Instead, prepare your own wholesome meals with a pinch of unrefined sea salt or crystal salt to bring out the flavour. It's good for you.

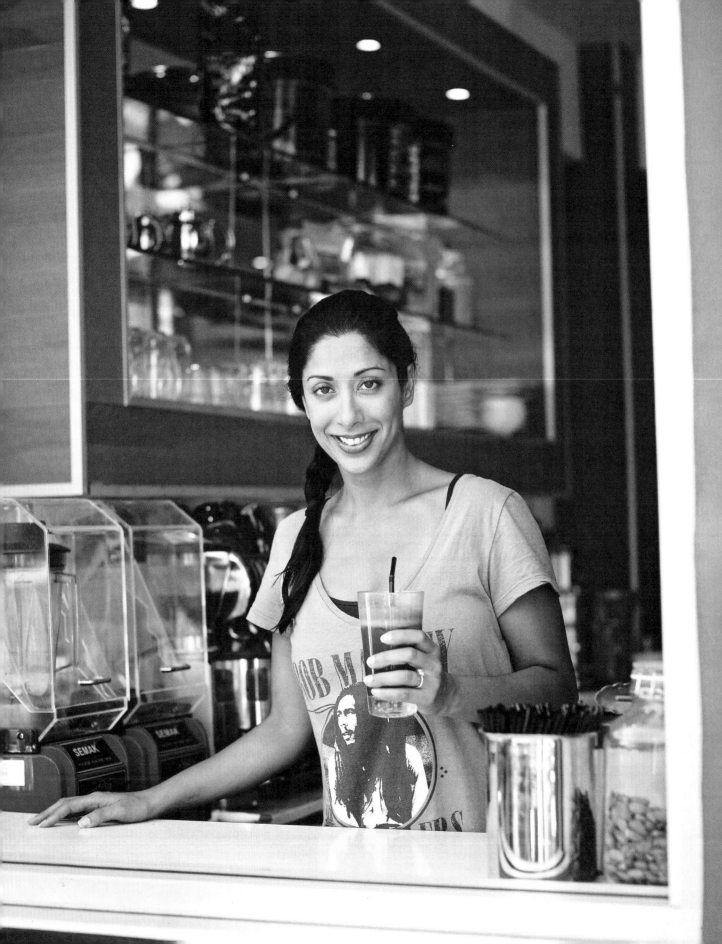

DETOXIFICATION

'The road to health is the one that begins
with an understanding and commitment to
cleanse and detoxify the body, to restore
balance, peace and harmony.'

— Dr Bernard Jensen

Detoxification is the ultimate anti-ageing tool. Naturopaths believe it's essential to
a healthy body, mind and spirit. It's the key to unlocking that youthful glow. It's the recipe for
boundless energy. Throughout history, people have fasted and cleansed their digestive systems,
and many religions feature a period of purification in their calendars: Judaism has Yom Kippur;
Islam has Ramadan; Jesus fasted for 40 days and nights, inspiring Lent.

You're probably asking, 'Why? Surely our bodies detoxify every day when we go to the toilet?'
Yes, your body has its own special elimination channels, specifically the bladder, bowel, liver,
kidneys, lungs and skin. But these organs can become over-burdened from overly acidic diets,
stress, low-grade food, the chemical-filled environments we often find ourselves in, and even
negative thinking. Unfortunately, in this day and age, we can accumulate far more toxins than
our elimination channels can handle.

Detoxification simply means helping the body to purge toxins that may have accumulated in
many different types of cells. By throwing out the 'garbage', you'll make your bodily processes
more effective. And detoxing from time to time will help your body cope when you do indulge
in a gourmet meal, fine wine or one too many Tim Tams.

In my clinical experience, the body shows signs of distress well before illness sets in. Signs
include headaches, backaches, lethargy, constipation, fatigue, bad breath, body odour, irritability,
depression, insomnia, confusion, skin problems, weight problems, cellulite, gas, bloating,
diarrhoea, sciatic pain, allergies . . . shall I go on? Many of these 'everyday' symptoms are caused
by the build-up of toxins. They're trying to tell you something: it's time for a detox.

DETOX TO LOSE FAT

Our fat cells exist to protect us. When more toxins are circulating than we can get rid of, natural medicine experts believe that we store them in our fat cells to protect us from them. This makes them difficult to get rid of, because our bodies are reluctant to let go of the fat cells that surround the toxin for fear that if released, it may cause us harm. However, when we detox, we signal to our bodies that it's okay to let go.

Detoxification is like taking your car in for a yearly service. It helps your body to fire on all cylinders. You need to allow your body the opportunity to heal itself so you can be your very best – inside and out. If weight loss is your goal, you can shave off a few centimetres with a detox, too. Bonus!

A SOLID FOUNDATION

You'll start with a 14-day detox diet that's designed to ignite your natural detoxification systems. It will overhaul your digestion, appearance, energy levels and mood. It will mean fewer trips to the doctor. It will transform the way you feel about yourself and how you present yourself to the world.

So, what does detoxification actually involve? Well, you won't starve or live off grapefruit and wheatgrass, I promise. You'll simply reduce your exposure to toxins and eliminate the toxins already lurking in your body. I'm prescribing you a healthy, holistic program accompanied by nourishing supplements and therapies. Here's why we should all detox, in a little more detail.

DETOX FOR YOUR LIVER

The liver is one of the most important organs of your body – and the biggest, at a whopping 1.5 kg. It filters toxins from the blood, converts carbohydrates from food into glucose for energy, breaks down proteins into amino acids and produces bile, which breaks down fats in the small intestine. It clocks extra hours when you ingest medications, by breaking them down into a usable form and eliminating the toxic waste products. The liver is often overworked and underpaid.

The simplest way to support your liver is to limit saturated fats, alcohol, sugary food, caffeine, carbonated drinks and over-the-counter drugs, and to eat more antioxidant-rich foods such as fruit, dark green leafy vegetables, herbs and spices, lots of fibre, brussels sprouts and broccoli, which also contain the cancer-fighting, antimicrobial compound, sulforaphane. Amino acids that support the liver include: arginine, taurine, methionine, glutamine and glutathione. Plants such as milk thistle, turmeric, globe artichoke, schisandra, yellow dock and dandelion root are little miracle workers. Getting enough high-quality water, soluble and insoluble fibre and good oils is critical to good liver health.

DETOX FOR THE KIDNEYS

The kidneys are responsible for excreting one to two litres a day of water via the urinary system. They balance the salts and acids in your body, while synthesising hormones such as the one that regulates blood pressure. It's important to look after them: according to Kidney Health Australia, one in three adults are at risk of kidney disease and a person can lose 90 per cent of kidney function before any symptoms develop. If you don't drink more than a litre of water per day, the mineral salt calcium oxalate can build up and eventually form a painful kidney stone.

Your kidneys also filter blood and can be burdened if a detoxification program is too rapid and intense. Support the kidneys by drinking pure water, plus cleansing herbal teas like nettle leaf, marshmallow root, juniper, parsley, red clover, goldenrod and clivers. To prevent kidney stones, up your potassium intake with a vegetable broth of celery, corn silk, barley or buchu. Other potassium-rich foods include cranberries, cherries, watermelon, pumpkin seeds, blueberries, bananas and asparagus. Magnesium and B-complex vitamins, especially B2 and B6, also aid the kidneys.

mind and body, help ward off diseases and eliminate toxins. And it costs you nothing.

Yogis call the breath *prana*, meaning 'life force'. They have a saying: 'Quality of breath is quality of mind.' Ever seen a stressed yogi? Yoga's one of the top ways to learn deep breathing, but if it's not for you, practise just 10 to 20 minutes of diaphragm breathing a day. Consider a meditation course. Correct breathing is non-negotiable. Get good at it and you'll look as amazing as you feel.

Lung foods include onions, garlic, apricots, almonds, pumpkin, thyme, cloves and parsley. And some of the best lung herbs include licorice root, marshmallow root, mullein, echinacea and thyme.

DETOX FOR THE LUNGS

Our lungs draw about 10,000 litres of air into our bodies every day, delivering oxygen to the bloodstream while expelling carbon dioxide. After the skin, lungs are the second line of defence against toxins, filtering pollutants from cars, factories, cleaning products, cigarette smoke, dirt, dust and mould. When the lungs are compromised – say, because of smoking or pneumonia – it's more difficult for our respiratory system to get the oxygen it needs and more toxins could infiltrate the bloodstream. Not exactly ideal.

Lung health is also marred by stress, anxiety and fast, shallow breathing. When we're wound up, it's easy to forget how to breathe properly. Fast 'chest' breathing kicks up your blood pressure, and high blood pressure (hypertension) can lead to heart attack, kidney failure and stroke. Practising deep breathing is an easy way to de-stress the

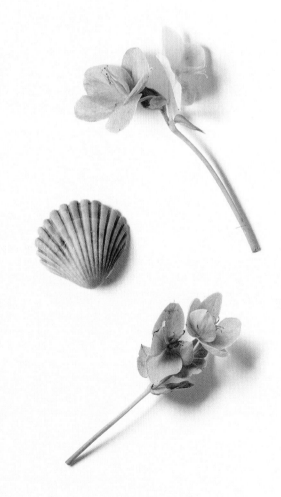

DETOX FOR THE COLON

The colon, bowel or large intestine is one of the most important elimination channels in the body and requires hydration and fibre to work at its best. Natural medicine experts believe that if we have an 'unclean' bowel, it doesn't matter how much good, clean food we take in because all this food does is sit on top of other undigested food and toxins and ferment. That is why when embarking on any health program, we must first detox the bowel.

And did you know that most of our immune system is found in the digestive tract? With a pH of between one and three, gastric acid in your stomach kills bacteria from food, while mucosal lining all through the tract forms a protective barrier against nasties. Helpful bacteria, known as 'gut flora', maintain order in the intestines and gut-associated lymphoid tissue (GALT) stores T and B lymphocytes (white blood cells), which attack foreign invaders. We have to keep our colons clean because the gut wall plays a vital part in the immune system, and it is our immune system which defends us against bacteria, microbes, viruses, toxins and parasites.

Some scientists even refer to the digestive tract as a 'second brain'. There is now a wealth of evidence showing a link between the mind, gut, emotions and immune responses in the body; there is a strong relationship between the state of our digestive systems and how we feel. What's more, 95 per cent of the body's serotonin – the happy hormone – is located in the gut (gut feeling, anyone?). All brilliant reasons why you need to maintain the health of your digestive tract.

Acidic foods and lifestyles adversely affect our colon's balance of gut flora (helpful bacteria), enabling parasites and candida albicans to run riot, causing an acidic environment and lowered immunity. Parasite and yeast overgrowth can make you vulnerable to illnesses from constipation to irritable bowel syndrome, bloating and even cancer. Naturopaths believe that detoxing the colon eliminates parasites, controls yeast growth and balances the beneficial micro-flora.

Gut flora is a trillion-strong community of good bacteria that eats away at undigested fibre, combats harmful bacteria and viruses, produces vitamins K and B, and more, in the colon. Healthy gut flora could decrease your likelihood of obesity. Basically, your colon has its own army. So it's important to protect and feed gut flora, especially if you're taking antibiotics, which are known to destroy it. Probiotics are the live cultures found in some yoghurt and fermented products such as kefir that help re-populate gut flora, while prebiotics are fodder for the probiotics and gut flora. Prebiotics include indigestible fibres such as those found in oats, banana, onion, leek, garlic and chicory.

DETOX FOR THE SKIN

Your skin is by far the largest organ of your body but it's often taken for granted. In Australia, we bask in the sun, slather random beauty products on our skin, dip it in dishwashing detergent and inject it with cosmetic treatments. Skin is a complex organ. It protects us from foreign microbes. It really matters what you put on your skin and how you treat it.

An easy way to detoxify the skin is dry brushing with a vegetable bristle brush before showering (see p 195). This stimulates the lymphatic system, enhances circulation and exfoliates dead skin cells. Follow with a warm shower or an Epsom salt bath. I also recommend bentonite clay and detoxifying oils (p 195).

Massage is pampering *and* therapeutic, improving circulation and lymph flow, relaxing tight muscles and de-stressing your body. All this, in turn, aids the detox process. Go one better: splash out on a detox wrap or salt scrub, which helps to accelerate the elimination of toxins. You'll feel on top of the world.

Feed your skin from the inside out, with foods rich in the antioxidants beta-carotene, zinc, and vitamins A, C and E. Include healthy monounsaturated fats such as avocado, olive and wheatgerm oils, and foods rich in silica (which minimises wrinkles by making collagen). Silica-rich foods include leafy green vegetables, cucumber, millet, oats, onions, rice, whole grains, alfalfa, barley and beetroot.

Replace posh lotions with cups of green tea and rosehip tea. Sweat a lot to clean skin cells. Jump in the ocean as often as possible. It's one of the best things you can do to recharge and revitalise your skin. The healing properties of the sea tone the skin, nourish the organs and increase blood circulation. If you can't get there, a salt bath (Epsom salt, sea salt or Himalayan crystal salt are my faves) is the next best thing.

DETOX FOR THE SPIRIT

Sure, it's great to cleanse your body. But detoxification is also about slowing down, relaxing and coming back to a sense of self. It's a time for reflection and contemplation, re-evaluating where you want to be and what 'stuff' you need to let go of. It's normal to feel angry, sad, teary, emotional or irritable in the first few days of a detox. When you detox your body, you also cleanse your mind and spirit. To paraphrase Sally Kempton, author of *Meditation for the Love of It*, think of these

emotions as clouds passing in the sky; watch them float past, rather than trying to catch and hold on to them. Negative or anxious thoughts no longer serve you, so let 'em go and make room for transformation and growth.

Eliminating stress and negativity is not only alkalising, it will boost your immunity, too. Scientists use the elaborate term 'psychoneuroimmunology': the study of the interaction between psychological processes and the nervous and immune systems of the human body. Some people call it the 'stress-disease connection'; stress has been linked to everything from hair loss and irritable bowel syndrome to cancer and even death. There's more to the mind than meets the eye.

DETOX BENEFITS

My clients have found that these include returning to a naturally optimum weight, and finding it easier to maintain a healthy weight without constant dieting. They experience dramatically increased feelings of vitality and wellbeing, and often find their appetite is smaller. The detox will help you hone your body's ability to choose the right foods. Your allergies and food intolerances may subside. You might report less congestion, inflammation and fermentation. You'll be armed against chronic diseases; your immune system will be stronger. Your cravings may disappear entirely. You'll be more positive.

When toxins are forced out of hiding and sent packing, you may experience headaches, nausea or fluey symptoms. Supportive treatments like colon therapy (see 'Colon Therapy', on p 22), scrubs and massage help, as do gentle exercise, stretching, writing your thoughts down and loads of sleep. In my clinical experience, once the toxins are excreted, people feel lighter and more lucid and lively. Vitality will replace the heaviness. You'll be left with bright, sparkling eyes, clear skin, a mega dose of radiance, and lots of energy to boot.

THE FINE PRINT

Ladies, if you're pregnant or breastfeeding, give detox a miss. Your body has other priorities. For everybody else, if you'd like to detox but are taking prescription meds or have a serious condition that requires monitoring, ensure you're supervised by a naturopath, or your health-care practitioner.

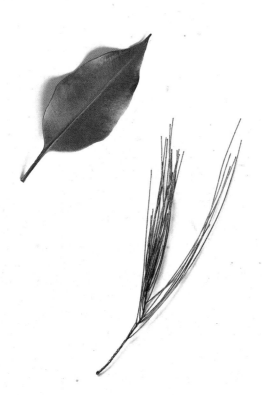

COLON THERAPY

Colon therapy is also known as a 'colonics', 'colon hydrotherapy', 'colon lavage' and 'colonic irrigation'. Proponents believe it flushes away toxins in order to achieve optimum health, beauty and lightness of being. Forms of colon therapy have been around for centuries – even the Greek historian Herodotus documented the enema, circa 440 BC.

Colon therapy simply involves hydrating the colon (large intestine) in a 45-minute session. The colon is gently infused with approximately 15 litres of warm, purified water, while a therapist uses massage and pressure-point techniques to work loose compacted faecal matter so it can be eliminated.

A word of warning: colon therapy is undergoing a resurgence in popularity, so there are cheaper, dodgy types of colonic therapies out there claiming to be 'the real thing'. One is the open system; another is the DIY colema board. Both of these methods are self-administered and work against the natural, in-built urge to pass bowel motions. You'll only ever hope to clean out your descending colon (one-third of your bowels) and it's much safer to opt for the closed system, executed entirely by a trained therapist.

I have written at length about colon therapy and its benefits on my website, www.thelastresort.com.au

| CASE STUDY |

ALEX DIMITRIADES, *actor*

I've always maintained a reasonable balance, and this I attribute to the teachings of my mother, who always provided the family with strong values of solid nutrition and, of course, the everlasting motto 'fresh is best'. No matter what else is going on in life, nutrient-rich foods are so important for wellbeing and health. Just as much as (if not more than) any other single element.

My daily routine changes all the time, but ideally would revolve around a morning swim in the ocean, followed by a fresh fruit breakfast, and then on with the day! In the course of a typical day, I'll eat lots of fresh produce, put together with reasonable level of expertise. I guess it helps growing up with good cooks in the family; no-one actually taught me anything, but by some mysterious process of osmosis, I rarely need to depend on processed foods as part of my diet. Caloric content aside, high preservative and low vitamin/mineral foods really don't deserve any place on the table. I try and avoid these things as much as possible, refined sugars especially! Also drinking plenty of water is essential.

I tend to go pretty easy on the exercise these days, probably due to overdosing in the gym as a teenager, but I have my moments. Avoiding injury is very important for me, so low-impact exercise suits me best. Swimming, soft sand runs, a few free weights. Rarely though. The inner healing nature of certain slow movements such as yoga and tai chi are something that interest me, but I think I need a little more practice.

To relax, I love nothing more than enjoying a nice afternoon on the beach with a gentle breeze blowing offshore, spraying the lip off the rolling crystal-clear swells, watching the sun set into the evening, followed by an amazing dinner of freshly caught chargrilled seafood and some nice wine. Of course none of this has the same significance without the aid of good company.

Health is a bank, and your body is the account. It's only as fruitful and abundant as that of the deposits and investments made. And that's not just nutrition-wise either; emotional and intellectual stimulation are also equally important. And we mustn't forget to laugh; the best medicine is so much fun!

To stay healthy, my top tip is to keep stress away. Impossible as it may seem, I believe it defines our health and longevity, ultimately. Much of this is also down to genetic predisposition, of course, but I certainly believe stress plays a major part.

Aussie lifestyle secrets come down to a laidback attitude and enjoying the fruits of the land the way nature intended. Being at one with the earth is something we all relate to here in our vast beautiful country, and it's certainly something to be envied, in my opinion.

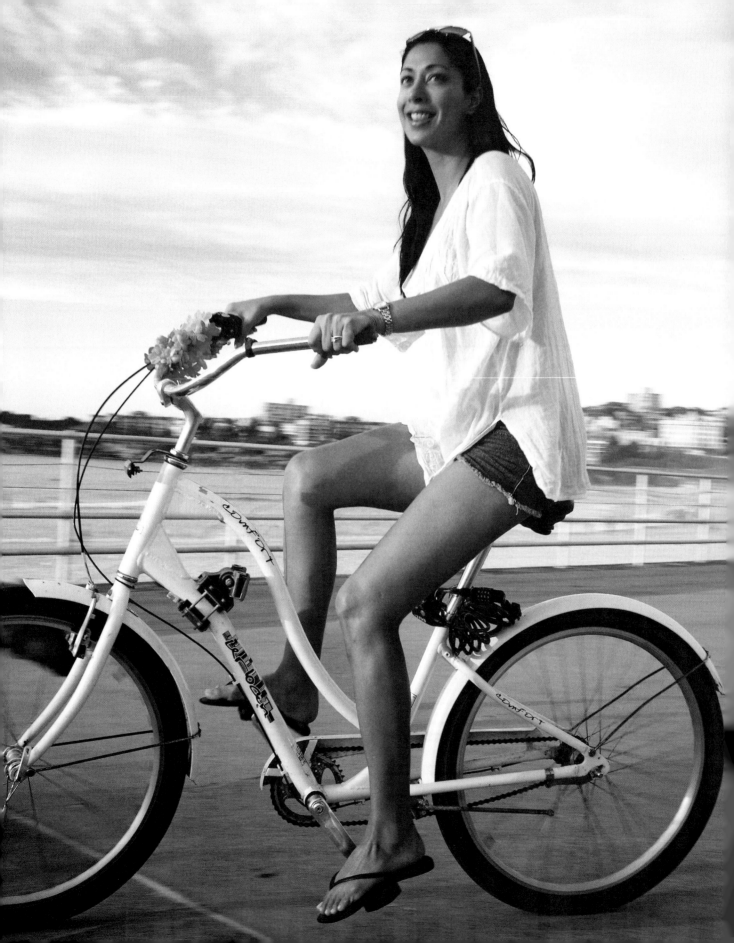

MOVEMENT

'No pain, no palm; no thorns, no throne;
no gall, no glory; no cross, no crown.'

— William Penn, 1682

Move it or lose it. We're designed to move, not sit at a desk all day. Movement eases tension, boosts circulation, stimulates the metabolism, releases endorphins, fires up the libido, wards off disease . . . the more you move, the more enriched your life will be. We all know how good exercise is for us, but we are so good at finding excuses *not* to do it. Exercise should be a habit, just like flossing or checking Facebook. There are no shortcuts; you can't outsource it. But regular exercise doesn't need to be a chore.

You don't need to log hours in the gym, running on the treadmill like a hamster on a wheel. And you don't need to pay a drill sergeant. Exercise can be anything you want it to be – the more varied the better. Just move your body. Some days you're itching to put on your sneakers; some days you'd rather defrost a fridge than exercise. I get it. Even on the difficult days, just try. Do something. Consistency is the key.

When you use your muscles for more than just lifting shopping bags, they increase in strength and size. They become less easily fatigued and work more efficiently. If you don't use your muscles enough, they can literally waste and everything becomes difficult. When you exercise, your heart – the most important muscle – works harder to pump blood around, as there's an increased need for oxygen. Your cardiovascular system becomes more efficient and better at circulating oxygen even when you're stationary. Everything becomes easier: climbing stairs, chasing after toddlers and, yep, carrying shopping bags.

CARDIO HEALTH

When we exercise, our hearts have to work more efficiently to pump the blood around as we need more oxygen for proper cell functioning. The more we exercise the more toned our cardiovascular systems become, circulating more oxygen even when we're not exercising. This naturally stimulates a feeling of wellbeing, as I believe oxygen is alkalising to the blood.

THE LYMPHATIC SYSTEM

The lymphatic system is a network of tiny vessels and a major part of the immune system. It removes excess fluid – called lymph – from the tissues of our body, stops off at lymph nodes where white blood cells attack bacteria, microbes and cancer cells, then returns the filtered lymph to the bloodstream. If the lymphatic system isn't working properly, a range of illnesses can develop, such as oedema, glandular fever and even Hodgkin's disease.

Unlike the bloodstream, the lymphatic system doesn't have a built-in pump: it relies solely on muscular contraction to move the lymph in one direction (towards the heart). If you don't move, the system breaks down. Activity, massage and dry skin brushing help to keep lymph moving.

YOUR BRAIN

Exercising not only helps with circulation, muscle growth and lymphatic drainage; it's essential for optimal cognitive function. When you work out, your blood transports more oxygen – food for your brain. In a study of 1.2 million Swedish men, fit twins scored higher IQs than their less-fit brothers. Exercise stimulates your brain to produce new neurons and repair damaged ones. Exercise is also strongly associated with a reduced risk of dementia as it slows down the age-related shrinkage of the frontal cortex, which is important for memory and recall.

The relationship between exercise and mood is now well documented. Exercise stimulates the release of neurotransmitters such as norepinephrine, serotonin, dopamine and endorphins – chemicals that significantly lift your mood. It makes you feel good. Researchers believe regular exercise can help treat depression. What's more, exercise stimulates our brains to produce new neurons and repair damaged ones, as well as to produce 'anti-ageing' hormones (dehydroepiandrosterone and growth hormone).

Exercise helps us achieve our very best, inside and out. If you want it to, exercise can push boundaries, increase pain threshold, and boost focus and tolerance. Overcoming physical challenges hones the mind. Top athletes are very determined characters because they constantly test their limits, make mindfulness part of their daily lives and never, ever give up.

WEIGHT LOSS

Movement is vital to weight loss. Nothing new here. You simply need to follow this equation: expend more energy than you take in. Exercise more, eat less. And if you build more muscle through weight-bearing and resistance exercises, you'll burn more kilojoules when you're doing nothing. Lucky for those of us who like to indulge!

If you diet but don't exercise, you'll still lose weight. But you'll shed muscle as well as fat and when you regain weight, it all comes back as fat. Every time you lose muscle through dieting, you reduce your ability to burn fat. It only gets harder and harder to fight the fat. Cardiovascular exercise is important for everybody, but especially relevant to weight loss. It means working up to 80 per cent of your maximum heart rate (your MHR is roughly 220 minus your age). So if you're running with a friend, you won't be chatting.

Staying active is essential for cardiovascular health, preserving and building muscle and losing excess lard. In turn, your self-esteem shines. I won't lie to you: it requires a bit of commitment and dedication. Make it easier on yourself by choosing an exercise schedule that suits your lifestyle. If you've got kids, play chasey in the park for an hour. If you loathe gyms, buy a Pilates DVD. If your schedule's busier than the Prime Minister's, cycle or walk to work. If you can incorporate exercise into your routine, it will give you so many gifts. Your brain will be clearer; you'll work smarter, not harder. You might even be able to leave work sooner and have more time for yourself. You might find you're less snappy at the kids or your partner thanks to those wonderful happy hormones. You'll feel more alive.

For optimum fitness, vary your type of sport, intensity and duration. Include conditioning as well as cardio. All athletes now incorporate some form of stretching or yoga as an essential part of their training. Yogis say, 'You can tell the age of a person by the flexibility of their spine', and it couldn't be more true – as we age, our bodies become more acidic, and acidity makes us rigid. Stretching and yoga are deeply alkalising as they aid in oxygenating tissue, whilst removing metabolic acids, preventing injuries and keeping us youthful to boot.

GOAL-SETTING

Goal-setting is like having a GPS when driving through unfamiliar territory – you'll have a much better chance of getting to your destination if you've thought about your goal and what it will take to get you there. To set meaningful goals, ask yourself:

What do you really want? Challenge yourself.

When do you want it? Be precise and set a specific time frame.

How will you get it? List at least 10 smaller, specific steps (such as finding a group to train with or getting a babysitter).

Why do you want it? Get personal here. Understanding why you really want it will help you achieve your goal.

Who will help you get there? Who can support you, motivate you and give you feedback?

Where is it taking you? Always fit your goals into your long-term vision.

When writing down your goals, make them **precise** and **positive**. And always **visualise** the thing you want to achieve in as much detail as you can. Unleash your imagination and run wild with it!

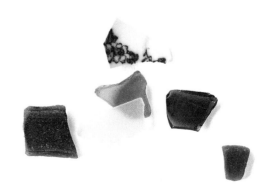

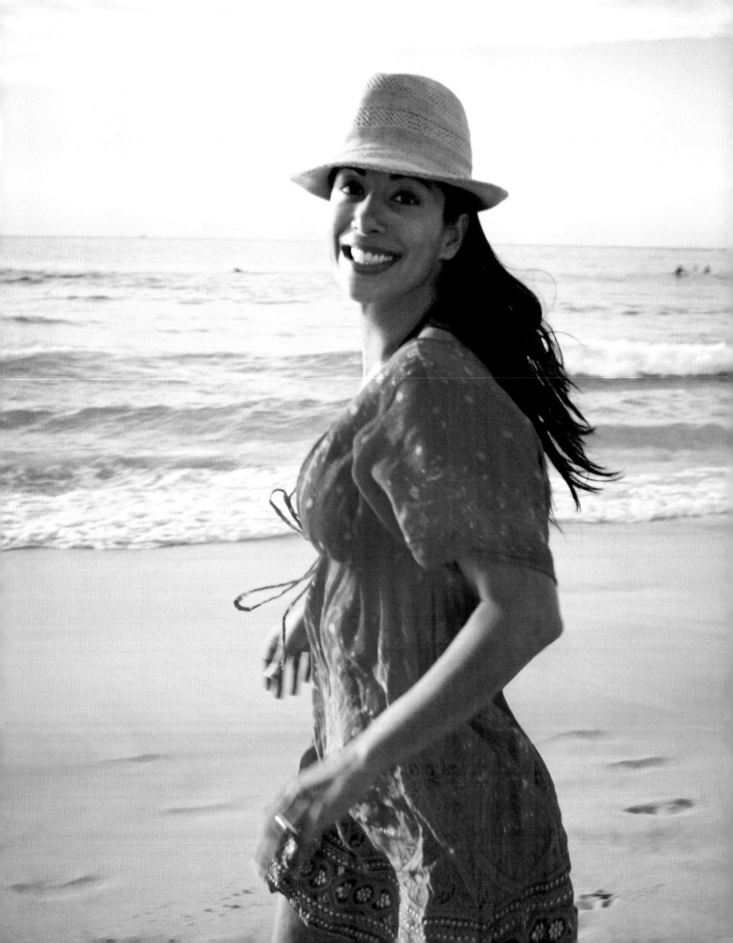

SUNLIGHT

Sunlight is a nutrient. Without it, there would be no plants, no Earth and no people. It's as crucial as oxygen, food or water. Exposing your skin to enough sunshine regularly is vital for optimal health – and your mindset. How do you feel after a 12-hour day in the office? Happy or haggard? Inspired or irritable? Sunlight makes us happy. (Sorry to be morbid for a second, but serotonin levels are often higher in the post-mortem brains of people who die in summer.) Yes, it's so important to be careful: skin cancer is a big risk in Australia. But all life on Earth is dependent on sunshine.

The sun provides essential vitamin D. Unless you've been living under a rock, you have probably heard that ultraviolet B (UVB) rays from sunlight synthesise vitamin D production – which is vital for calcium absorption from our food. Adequate calcium means stronger bones. If you don't get enough vitamin D, brittle bones and rickets can occur; one of the primary reasons bones become brittle in the elderly is a lack of sun exposure.

Vitamin D deficiency has been linked with multiple sclerosis, glandular fever and gestational diabetes. Sunlight, or UVB light therapy, is often prescribed to treat the skin conditions eczema and psoriasis – my patients have found it extremely beneficial for these glandular disturbances of the skin. Moreover, a lack of vitamin D can lead to poor immune function, which may be why we're more susceptible to colds and viruses in winter than summer.

You can get some vitamin D from foods such as oily fish (sardines, mackerel, salmon, tuna), eggs and mushrooms, but health experts agree the sun's rays are the best source. Obviously, roasting yourself isn't the answer (sorry, tan fans). You only need to expose your face, arms and hands for 10 to 15 minutes a day; in the early morning or late afternoon during summer, of course!

The rule of thumb is the darker you are, the more sunlight you require to activate your body's ability to synthesise Vitamin D.

Sunlight directly affects our red blood cell count. If you don't get enough sunlight, you can become anaemic. But with sufficient sunlight, the blood's ability to carry oxygen is increased, your circulation improves, and consequently your immune function and its ability to repair and rebuild tissue is increased.

Sunlight influences the size and strength of our muscles, and enhances their ability to contract by improving the condition of the entire body, including the nerves that control the muscles. A lack of sunlight can lead to muscle atrophy.

Natural medicine experts also believe that sunlight also directly affects the levels of acid in our bodies; enough full-spectrum sunlight helps you maintain alkalinity; without it, your immune system, skin vitality, vitamin D production and so on are compromised.

Your circadian rhythm needs sunlight. Known as your 'body clock' or 'internal clock', circadian rhythms influence your sleep patterns and your metabolism. Inside your hypothalamus in the brain is a mass of nerve cells called the suprachiasmatic nucleus (SCN). This is a master clock set to a 24-hour schedule that tells you when to wake up, when to eat and when to go to bed – your circadian rhythm.

We humans are diurnal creatures – we're awake during sunlight hours. Every time you wake up, stretch and see daylight, your SCN gets the message to reset your circadian rhythm. This kick-starts various hormone and enzyme secretions. For example, levels of the stress hormone cortisol peak between 6 and 8 a.m., making you feel awake and hungry.

In the evening after the sun goes down, cortisol drops and 'the hormone of darkness', melatonin, rises – reducing your appetite and making you calm and sleepy. According to researchers, short sleep duration leads to low levels of leptin (a hormone that suppresses appetite) and high levels of ghrelin (which stimulates appetite). If you work with your body's circadian rhythm, you can maintain your sleep quality and tap into your natural hunger cues, staving off weight gain.

GET YOUR BEAUTY SLEEP

Establish a regular bedtime routine. Wind down so you're ready to hit the sack between 9 and 11 p.m. Brush your teeth, don the PJs, read a book. Rise at the same time every day, even if you've had a bad night's sleep.

Switch off, literally. Studies show that artificial light, and computer and TV screens, may inhibit the body's production of melatonin, making it harder to fall asleep.

Get 20 minutes of sunlight first thing. Sleep specialists reckon this is the best way to reset your circadian clock if you're suffering from insomnia. Exercise at the same time for double the benefits.

Eat more during daylight hours and less at night. Work with your biochemical rhythm, increasing your ability to digest and metabolise food. You'll experience fewer cravings late in the evening.

Avoid alcohol after 9 p.m. You might think it helps you relax into some 'me time', but alcohol can disturb sleep patterns. It might be boring but a chamomile, passionflower or valerian-infused herbal tea is way more effective.

| CASE STUDY |

JESSICA GOMES, *international model*

When I was young my mother looked after me very well and taught me to eat healthily. But when I reached 17, I hit a rebellious stage. Then when I moved to New York and started taking my career seriously, I got into the whole holistic and organic way of life. Now I would say I'm at a happy medium, and Saimaa's program has helped me achieve this.

Right now I dance every day (for Korean *Dancing with the Stars*) and I eat six small meals a day. I take an algae supplement, fish oil and magnesium at night; I also have a lot of good fats and high protein in my diet. I try to keep as active as possible with my busy schedule. And have lots of water!

My diet consists of organic meat, fish and vegetables. Some carbs, whether it's brown bread or rice. I like eggs in the morning and I snack on fruit and nuts. No alcohol, except maybe some wine on special occasions, and lots of green tea and water. One coffee a day is my rule.

My favourite forms of exercise are dancing, boxing and weights, and to relax I have massages and treat myself to detox retreats. You just have to do what works for you and what makes you happy. Do what you feel is right. Keep it simple and trust yourself. Also it's about having common sense and it must be realistic for your needs. I say, think back to how Adam and Eve lived!

The best tips I can offer for staying healthy are: don't smoke or drink – simple! And think about where your food comes from. Eat whole foods. Beach and sun keep people happy and healthy. And try to lead a simple life – avoid too much stress and worry.

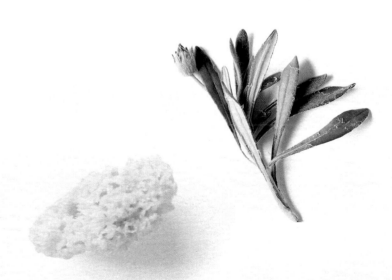

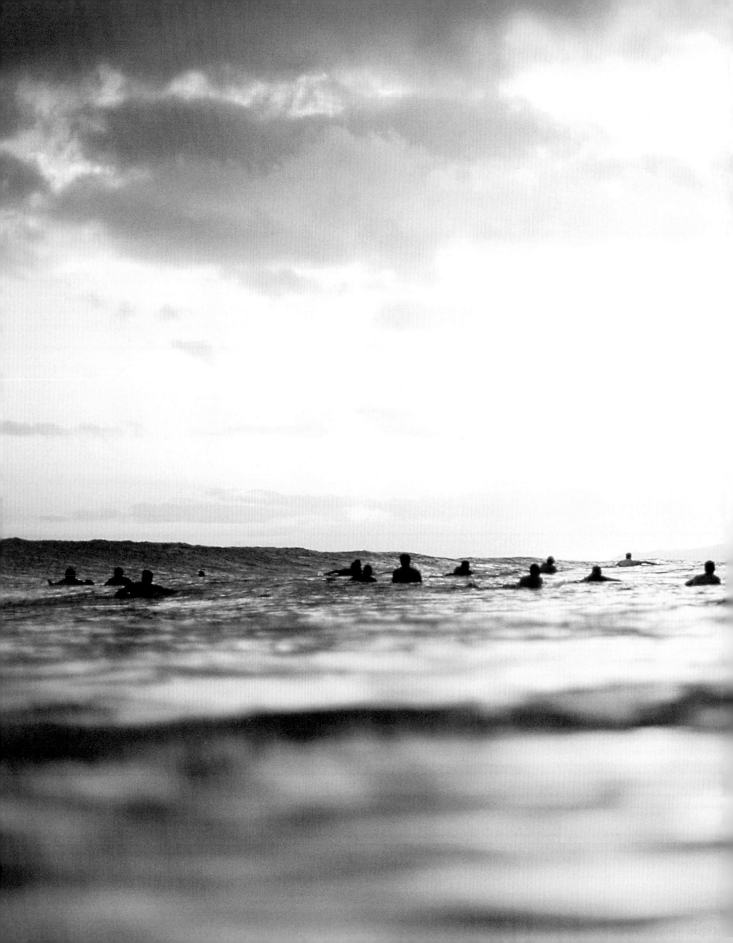

POSITIVITY

'The thought manifests as the word;
the word manifests as the deed,
the deed develops into habit;
and the habit hardens into character.
So watch the thought and its ways with care;
and let it spring from love born out of
concern for all beings.
As the shadow follows the body,
as we think, so we become.'

— From the *Dhammapada, Awakening the Buddha Within*
by Lama Surya Das

Thoughts create your destiny. And attitude steers it. Our outlook determines how we think, how we act and therefore how our lives unfold. Maintaining a positive outlook is something only you can do – and it's just as imperative to our health as nutrition, exercise or sunlight. If you think, 'I'm never going to do such-and-such,' you won't! Your happiness or unhappiness can depend on the approach you take to life.

Sure, some things are out of our control. But think of some everyday miracles in life, like two people deciding to start a family. Very soon the product of that one thought is a beautiful child. Slightly less miraculously, ever find that on the days you're in a foul mood, everything goes wrong?

The way you *perceive* things can also have a powerful effect on what happens next. The Dalai Lama said, 'Although you may not always be able to avoid difficult situations, you can modify the extent to which you suffer by how you choose to respond to the situation.' Or, in layperson's terms, you can cry or you can laugh. Stress, for example, isn't an external force that controls your behaviour – it is a response to the situation determined by how you perceive it.

And stress can be dangerous. Stress can betray our bodies from the inside, lowering immunity and making us more susceptible to colds and flu. Natural medicine experts believe this is due to the simple fact that stress causes acidity in our bodies. At its worst, prolonged stress can cause heart disease, which we all know can lead to heart attack and stroke. (More on stress in the next chapter.) Positivity, on the other hand, can save your life. A University of Pittsburgh study found that people over 50 who 'saw the glass as half-full' (versus half-empty) were 30 per cent less likely to die from heart disease.

In Ayurvedic medicine, the name for toxin is 'ama' and it refers to either a physical or mental toxin. Thoughts and emotions are powerful forces that can alter our internal chemistry. Nutrition and exercise help, but you can only be so healthy if you're thinking acidic thoughts. Eliminate the ama by changing your attitude towards whatever's worrying you. Learn to see the positive side of a situation and resist the urge to complain or speak ill of others.

Don't let your history define you.
Negative thoughts – anger, sadness, frustration – can manifest in your physical health. But you have the power to free yourself of emotional malaise. We all have a story about where we came from and how it influences our behaviour. You can choose to allow pain, hate or regret to eat away at your soul and wellbeing, or decide that your past isn't who you are. It's your attitude to life that defines you. Find a way to let go of bad memories and if someone's wronged you, find a way to forgive the person. You'll feel at peace. Forgiveness doesn't mean condoning bad behaviour – it's about freeing yourself from negativity.

In the words of the artist and poet Kahlil Gibran, 'Beauty is not in the face, it is a light in the heart.' Your attitude towards yourself, others, life and stressors can make you more (or less) beautiful. Self-esteem peaks when you love who you are and feel confident in your choices. There is far more to beauty than simply the way you look. A positive attitude is the spark that makes you attractive.

I believe positivity – and compassion – is inherent in us all. You just have to observe human kindness and the natural beauty surrounding us. Embrace opportunities, appreciate the people that bring you joy and treat your body with love by giving it the correct fuel. It's also very true that practising 'random acts of kindness' – from smiling at strangers to volunteering – helps nurture a positive attitude.

Face your fears.
The nervous system is designed to take notice when you feel threatened: the 'fight or flight response'. It's nature's way of helping you get out of stressful or dangerous situations to reach safety quickly, by stimulating hormones such as adrenaline, noradrenaline and cortisol. But it's supposed to be for emergencies. It was really useful for the odd occasion in the cave-dwelling days but these days, stress is 'normal' and fear is omnipresent: fear of commitment, fear of rejection, fear of failure, even fear of success. These kinds of fear often stem from a belief that we're not good enough. It also lets you off the hook. Your brain comes up with all sorts of clever tricks – such as fear – to talk itself out of having to work hard. You can be your own best friend or worst enemy. You can meet challenges head-on or hide in a corner – it's up to you.

Ever found that when you've faced something you thought was terrifying, it wasn't as bad as you'd anticipated? Fear occurs when we care more about the goal than about the process. Overcoming fear is about having faith in yourself; see the process as beneficial, whatever the outcome. Moving out of your comfort zone and transcending your fears is so exhilarating – *that's* winning. A mistake is only a mistake if you don't learn from it.

Who cares what other people think?

It's a waste of creative energy worrying about people judging or not liking you. You can't control how people see you. No matter how wonderful you are, you will never be liked by everybody. Do you warm to everyone you meet? Bet you the answer is no! If people unfairly criticise you or talk about you behind your back, it comes from their own fear and insecurity. Your attitude is within your control. Don't stoop to their level. Try to be humble and compassionate, and maintain that positive outlook.

Meditation: not just for hippies. You

don't need to spend mega-bucks on a self-help course or erect a tepee. Meditation takes practice, but it's free and invaluable. It gives you mental space, calms the incessant chatter inside your head and allows you to just exist. The stillness lets you observe negative emotions and let them go. Meditation improves your emotional and physical health, while helping you discover your true nature.

You can meditate the traditional way, sitting upright and focusing on the breath, a mantra or an image. But if this doesn't suit you, don't despair. Meditation is all about mindfulness. It's being in 'the zone'. Meditation can happen when you're at one with your camera, trying to take that perfect shot, or catching the last barrel wave of the day. It's shushing the chatter and being 100 per cent in the act of what you're doing. That's it. The only thing that matters is right here, right now. Practise this often and, voilà, you'll be a meditator.

So let's end this chapter with this thought. You might have struggled with your beginning, things might have been tough, but that does not have to define who you are. So who do you choose to be? You choose the story of your life.

AFFIRM YOURSELF

Affirmations are positive statements you say to encourage yourself. You can make up your own or get them from a book – it doesn't matter. I swear by them. When said out loud, deliberately and daily, positive self-talk helps to stimulate brain chemistry and convince the brain it is ready to strive for your desired goal. Affirmations are the easiest and cheapest tool you can use to let go of limiting beliefs, replacing them with positive ones.

Write your goals down. Now, write down how you feel about these goals. Can you see them happening? What words pop into your head? For example, you might want to find your life partner or lose ten kilograms, but you might only hear things like. 'No one ever likes me' or 'I will never be slim.' Now, write down an affirmation beside each goal, such as 'I am lovable' or 'I will reach my happy weight.' If you are diligent and recite your affirmations every day, your brain starts believing you're already there.

Repeat your affirmations at least ten times every day. Morning is best as it starts you on the right foot for the day ahead. Very soon you'll find you're acting in line with your affirmations, getting closer to your goal, simply because you've talked yourself into it.

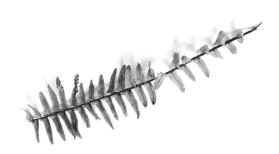

NATURE

We live in an age when unnecessary things
are our only necessities.

— Oscar Wilde

What have we done to our environment? Our culture of excessive consumption has
affected our planet in a very real and detrimental way. With the global financial crisis, followed
by the economic downturn in Europe, many of us are taking a step back and looking at how
much money and how many material things we actually need. There's a real movement towards
greener living because more 'stuff' doesn't make us happier. It can all be taken away. It may be
a cliché, but it's the simple things in life that put a smile on your dial. Spending time in nature
is one of those things.

Stress is a killer, as we discussed in the last chapter. It's easy to think stress is the natural
by-product of a modern, fast-paced lifestyle, but it doesn't have to be. There is an optimal
amount of stress, known as 'eustress', which is a positive force that helps us take up the
challenges life throws at us. It helps you burn the candle at both ends when you need to, or do
all your gift-shopping on Christmas Eve. Just as the fight or flight response helped us run from
sabre-toothed tigers thousands of years ago, that explosion of adrenaline helps get the job done.
But feeling stressed for prolonged periods? That's about as helpful as a boat in the desert.

Relaxing in a natural environment releases the mind and body. It's the quickest way
to de-stress. It allows you to be more present, calmer and happier. From walking the dog to
scaling a cliff-face (if that's your thing), nature does so much for your sense of self and is a vital
part of getting that Aussie Body. It allows you to focus on the little things, like sand between
your toes or the smell of eucalyptus – instead of deadlines or some snooty comment made by
a colleague. Spending time in nature also makes us humble and offers perspective; you realise
how insignificant you are in the bigger scheme of things (I mean that in a good way, like
appreciating the power of the ocean when you're being annihilated by a set of waves). There
are much greater forces out there.

On a physiological level, you breathe in more oxygen outdoors – unless of course you're hanging out by a freeway – and as we know, oxygen is incredibly nourishing to all the cells in the body. Money can't buy that. Studies show that people in proximity to green spaces live longer; even office plants contribute to greater feelings of wellbeing and decreased stress and fatigue. Urban life has a marked and permanent effect on our brains. According to research published in the journal *Nature*, city dwellers have a much higher risk of developing anxiety and mood disorders such as schizophrenia, compared with those who live in the country. In the brains of city-slickers, there's increased activity in the amygdala, the area of the brain that's stimulated during periods of stress.

Slow down and be 'bored'.

Boredom is the new luxury. Too many of us have diaries chock-a block with errands, catch-ups, kids' co-curricular activities, appointments . . . We put in extra hours at work so maybe we'll get a pay rise or promotion. We lose hours on social networking sites. Sound familiar? How often do you really have the opportunity to switch off, relax and savour some contemplation time? For five minutes at the end of yoga class? Just before you collapse into bed? It's not enough, frankly.

It's really no wonder that stress is one of our biggest killers. We don't give ourselves downtime. Did you know that, on average for any given year, Aussies have 123 million hours of accrued annual leave? Instead of taking time out, we're spurred on to do more, be more, have more, consume more. It's as if you're nobody unless you're super-busy! And it's so easy to be envious of others who have more than you. Next time you find yourself channelling the green-eyed monster, ask yourself, 'Is the person really any happier?' 'Is he/she any healthier?' 'Is the person

fulfilled or just busy?' True health and happiness really comes from 'less is more'.

So, switch off your mobile phone regularly and take breaks that don't involve the internet or television. Spend time on your own. It's a wonderful healing activity that helps you return to your true nature, your sense of self.

Let's do our bit.

Preserving the environment means we – and our children – can reap the bountiful benefits of nature for years to come. We live on the driest continent on Earth, so spend less time in the shower. We live in one of the sunniest countries on the planet so invest in solar energy to reduce your fuel costs. Switch off appliances at the wall and don't drive if you can walk or bike. Switch to a green energy provider. I could go on and on, but the most important way to protect the environment is to consume less. Don't buy stuff if you know it's going to end up in landfill. Eat organic and locally sourced produce when you can. You know the old adage: 'Think globally, act locally.' If we want to create change in the world, it has to start with us.

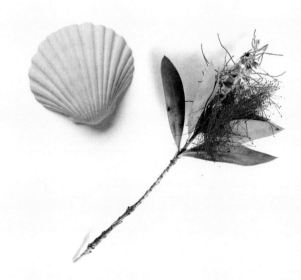

TECHNOLOGY AND RADIATION

The electronic devices we use most commonly, like mobile phones and computers, emit a small amount of radiation every time you talk, text or update your status. While the health risks haven't yet been confirmed, we know that radiation isn't exactly good, and could give rise to cancerous tumour growth in the body. A study of more than 13 000 Danish children found those who were exposed to mobile phones were 80 per cent more likely to have behavioural problems.

We're hooked on technology. We're almost all reliant on computers and mobile phones. Until we know for sure the effect they're having on us, it's best to minimise radiation exposure.

- Switch off devices at night – and really try not to sleep within a metre of any device or equipment.

- Consider texting more, using a hands-free kit or – gasp! – picking up the landline phone.

- Only make calls when there's ample coverage, otherwise your phone will emit more radiation as it as to work harder.

- Scientists have a theory that because children's heads are smaller, their skulls are thinner and they'll be using mobiles for longer than us, their brains are more sensitive to radiation. So limit their time on mobiles and tablets when their brains are developing.

- Consider buying a Tesla plate or an Aulterra neutraliser, which can rebalance the energy of your home and combat radiation. An anti-radiation holographic disc may also reduce or neutralise the harmful effects of electromagnetic waves.

| CASE STUDY |

SAMANTHA HARRIS, *supermodel*

Growing up, like any other kid, I did love the fast food but as I got older both my body and mind knew it didn't agree with me. I am fortunate to have a very supportive boyfriend who is very healthy and active. He's inspired me to be fit and healthy and I've never looked back.

My daily routine is to get up early, around 5 a.m., go to the gym, do my workout, come home, have breakfast and get ready for whatever the day may hold for me, whether it's a photoshoot, fashion show or castings.

I enjoy many types of exercise, and especially love high-impact classes at the gym. I do also love going for runs outdoors. My favourite way to relax is going out for a nice dinner somewhere with my boyfriend. I believe that what you put into your body shows on the outside and that it's really important to stay active.

My best lifestyle tip is: live life to the fullest and be happy with who you are. Never compare yourself to anybody because you're beautiful and unique in your own way.

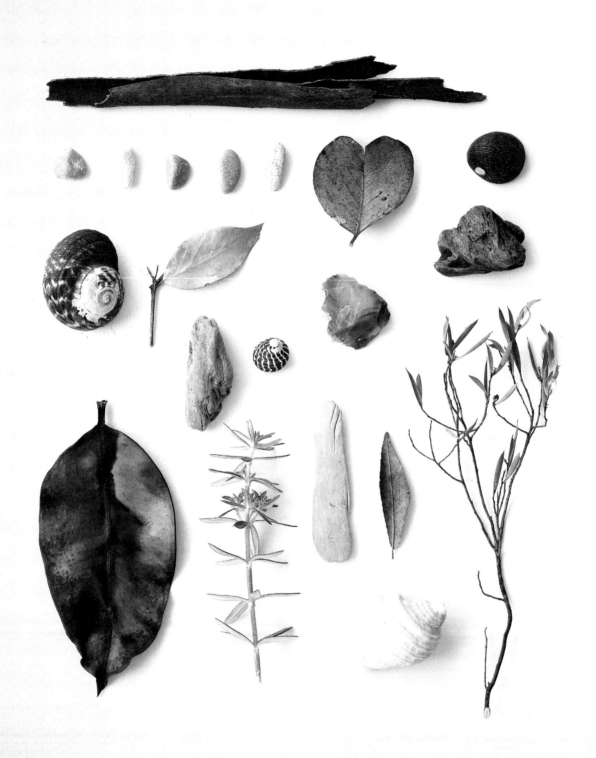

PART TWO

AUSSIE BODY
14-DAY DIET

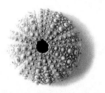

'When diet is wrong medicine is
of no use. When diet is correct
medicine is of no need.'

— Ayurvedic proverb

The Aussie Body 14-Day Diet is really a detox plan. This is the fun bit. By following this super-easy program, you'll feel brighter, lighter and more energetic. You will think more clearly. Friends will notice your radiant skin. You might feel 10 years younger. You'll feel more positive. And the rewards are yours in just two weeks.

Sure, you will probably lose some excess baggage, but this isn't just about 'dieting'. Most diets are painfully restrictive and bloody boring. Next time someone tells you they're only eating protein, only eating baby food or surviving on ground African mangoes and laxatives, ask yourself: do they look healthy? Are they glowing? Are they happy, calm and relaxed, with a lightness of being?

No, no and no. When people embark on prohibitive diets, they usually do lose weight. But they can look tired and drawn, their skin becomes congested and they sport dark circles under their eyes no amount of make-up can fix. Moreover, they tend to be grumpy and irritable. They can't think clearly. Their bodies and minds are crying out for nutrients!

What's more is that most of the weight that is lost comes from water and muscle mass instead of fat. Low energy (or kilojoule) intake forces the body to enter starvation mode and hang on to the existing fat for survival; if you deprive yourself, your metabolism actually slows down. And unfortunately, once you start eating normally again, you'll put the weight right back on.

The Aussie Body Diet is an entirely different approach. It's designed to help you achieve optimal wellbeing, reach a happy (not unhealthy) weight and have you feeling the best you've ever felt in your life. It will reignite your physiological intuition: your body will tell you what it needs, how much it needs, and when to eat, exercise and rest. It will decelerate the visible effects of ageing. You might find that your aches, pains and niggling symptoms disappear. You'll feel better about yourself and be kinder to others (yes, a 'diet' can do that). You'll have abundant, sustained energy. You'll look forward to exercising because it's easier to move your body. You'll feel happier, calmer and less foggy. In short, you'll be the very best you — inside and out! Not only that, you'll be saving thousands of dollars – preventing disease is a lot cheaper than curing it.

The Aussie Body 14-day Diet is based on traditional naturopathic principles designed to get the body motoring at top speed. They're centuries-old techniques – nothing new or scary – to clean the body of acidity, toxins and pathogens such as candida albicans. It's a holistic program, which means treating not just the body, but also the mind. Nourishing your cognitive, emotional and spiritual self is essential for true, long-lasting health – particularly in the fast-paced, materialistic and polluted world we live in.

Detoxification is vital. It cuts through chemical overload and cleanses your vital organs, from your liver, kidneys and bowel, to your skin and grey matter. I truly believe it's the easiest, most effective and quickest way to optimal health and sustainable weight loss.

Before you start, check in with yourself and note any ailments that are troubling you. You can use the Symptoms Questionnaire I've created online at www.aussiebodydiet. com. Refer to this each week, as it will help you monitor your progress. It's a fantastic motivational tool. Also, use the checklist (in Guides and Tools on p 194), to make sure you're utilising the lifestyle secrets discussed in Part One. Write down any therapies you're having or supplements you're taking. The Weekly Planner will help you form and maintain positive habits, and keep on top of all the wonderful, proactive steps you're taking towards achieving optimal health.

Note: this program isn't recommended in pregnancy, and if you suffer from a debilitating condition, are addicted to a harmful substance, take prescription medication or have serious health concerns, seek advice from your own naturopath or health practitioner before you start.

If you smoke cigarettes, it's better to use nicotine patches during the detox, as they eliminate your exposure to cancer-causing tar and nasty carbon monoxide. As you progress, you can reduce the nicotine amount per patch (eg from 15 mg to 10 mg, then 5 mg).

N.B. If you truly want to stop smoking or using any other substance, the Aussie Body Diet will help you to get you there, as on a physical level, the more you alkalise the body and clean the addiction from your system, the less likely you will feel the need to smoke or take harmful substances. And mentally, you will feel clearer about why you do it, using goal-setting to monitor your progress and remind you of how far you've come.

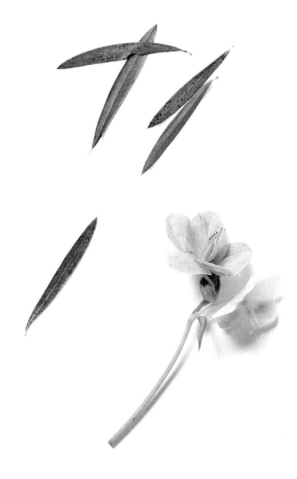

WHAT YOU'LL NEED TO AVOID
Gluten-containing grains for Detoxification Phase (Week 1); wheat in Nutritive Phase. You can have gluten-containing grains (except wheat) in second week (Nutritive Phase). These include rye, oats, spelt and barley.
Potatoes
Refined sugar
Alcohol
Caffeine and decaffeinated beverages. You can have up to two cups of green tea before midday each day.
Dairy products. Natural cow's yoghurt, plain Greek yoghurt, organic sheep or goat's milk yoghurt and cheese, and kefir are allowed.
Soy or soy products (exception is organic raw miso)
Corn and maize products
Red meat (for Detoxification Phase). Limit red meat to organic lamb in Nutritive Phase, which you can have up to three times per week.
Processed foods e.g. carbonated drinks, condiments such as tomato sauce, soy sauce, barbecue sauce, etc, and anything with preservatives or tinned (exception is tuna in water and some beans/legumes).
Vinegar and vinegary foods such as olives and pickles.
High-mould foods such as mushrooms and peanuts.
Oils and margarine substitutes, other than those listed in the table opposite.
Shellfish and crustaceans

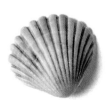
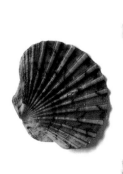
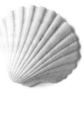
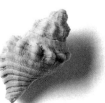

WHAT YOU CAN EAT	
Vegetables	Asparagus, beet greens, beetroot, bok choy, broccoli, brussels sprouts, cabbage, capsicum, carrots, cauliflower, celery, chicory, chilli, comfrey, cucumber, dandelion greens, eggplant, fennel, green beans, kale, leeks, lettuce, mustard greens, okra, onion, parsley, radish, rocket, silverbeet, snow peas, spinach, spring onions, sprouts (eg mung bean, sunflower and alfalfa), squash, swiss chard, tomato, watercress, witlof and zucchini.
Fruit	Limit to two small pieces of high-nutrient fruit per day: apples, kiwi fruit, lemon, lime, pears, pawpaw, pineapple, or a handful of berries. No more than one small banana or 1 tbsp shredded coconut, raisins, sultanas or dates per day. No more than one small avocado per day. N.B. try not to eat fruit directly after main meals.
Fish	Only blue-eyed trevalla, flathead, mackerel, mullet, salmon or sardines. If choosing tinned fish, make sure it's in water or olive oil (drained). N.B. in the second week, all types of fish except big-eyed tuna, swordfish and shark are allowed.
Meat	Chicken and turkey (breast and thigh only; no skin allowed; organic only). In second week, organic lamb is allowed.
Gluten-free grains	Amaranth, basmati rice, black bean 'spaghetti', brown rice, buckwheat, millet, montina (Indian rice grass), quinoa, red rice, sorghum, teff and wild rice. N.B. in second week, rye, oats, barley and spelt are ok.
Herbs, spices and seasonings	Basil, cardamom pods, cayenne pepper, Celtic salt, cinnamon, coriander, cumin, dulse, fennel, garlic, ginger, Himalayan pink rock salt, kelp, kombu, mint, nori, onion, parsley, red chilli, rosemary, sea salt flakes, turmeric, vegetable salts such as Herbamare, and wakame.
Condiments	All-purpose seasoning such as Bragg's, coconut water, dukkah, gomasio (a Japanese condiment made from sesame seeds and salt), raw apple cider vinegar, raw cacao, raw miso, tahini, home-made hummus, and tamari. 1 teaspoon of agave syrup, brown rice syrup or raw honey per day.
Beans and legumes	Adzuki, butter beans, cannellini, haricot, lima, navy beans, red kidney, lentils and black beans.
Eggs	Organic and free-range only; no more than six per week.
Dairy and milk substitutes	Only natural or Greek yoghurt, sheep milk and goat's milk yoghurt and cheese. Only raw, organic cultured dairy i.e. kefir. Use almond, hazelnut, oat, quinoa, rice and seed milks instead of dairy milk.
Nuts and seeds (maximum 20, whole and preferably soaked, or 2 tablespoons seeds).	Almonds, brazil nuts, cashews, chia seeds, flaxseed and linseed meal, hazelnuts, hemp seeds, pepitas (pumpkin seeds), sesame seeds, sunflower seeds and tahini.
Oils	Avocado oil, coconut oil, extra virgin olive oil, flaxseed oil or omega 3, 6 and 9 oil blend (do not heat these), hemp seed oil and sesame oil.
Herbal teas	Burdock, chamomile, echinacea, elderflower, fennel, ginger, gingko, green tea (2 cups before midday only), lemon, licorice, nettle, organic chai, peppermint, rosehip and St John's Wort.

AUSSIE BODY DETOX SHOPPING LIST

- Water filter (I recommend an ionised filter such as Bluezone Water)

- Fruit (see table on p 45 for specific types)

- Vegetables (see table on p 45 for specific types)

- Sprouts

- Herbs and spices (see table on p 45 for specific types), especially cayenne pepper

- Nuts and seeds (see table on p 45 for specific types)

- Oil (see table on p 45 for specific types)

- Protein – organic chicken, turkey, fish, beans, legumes, lentils (and lamb if desired in second week)

- Natural or Greek yoghurt, sheep milk and goat's milk yoghurt and cheese

- Raw, unfiltered organic apple cider vinegar

- Organic raw honey or agave syrup; and raw cacao 'chocolate'

- Coconut water

- Organic raw miso

- Brown rice cakes or crackers; 100 per cent rye crackers (if desired in Nutritive phase)

- Kefir

- Rice, almond, oat, quinoa or hazelnut milk (make sure these do not contain added sugar, including maltodextrin)

- Organic herbal tea including green tea (limit to two cups before midday), peppermint, fennel, nettle, ginger, lemon, elderflower, chamomile, licorice, organic chai, rosehip, detox blend, etc

- Gluten-free grains (see table on p 45 for specific types). (Rye, barley, oats and spelt if desired in second week)

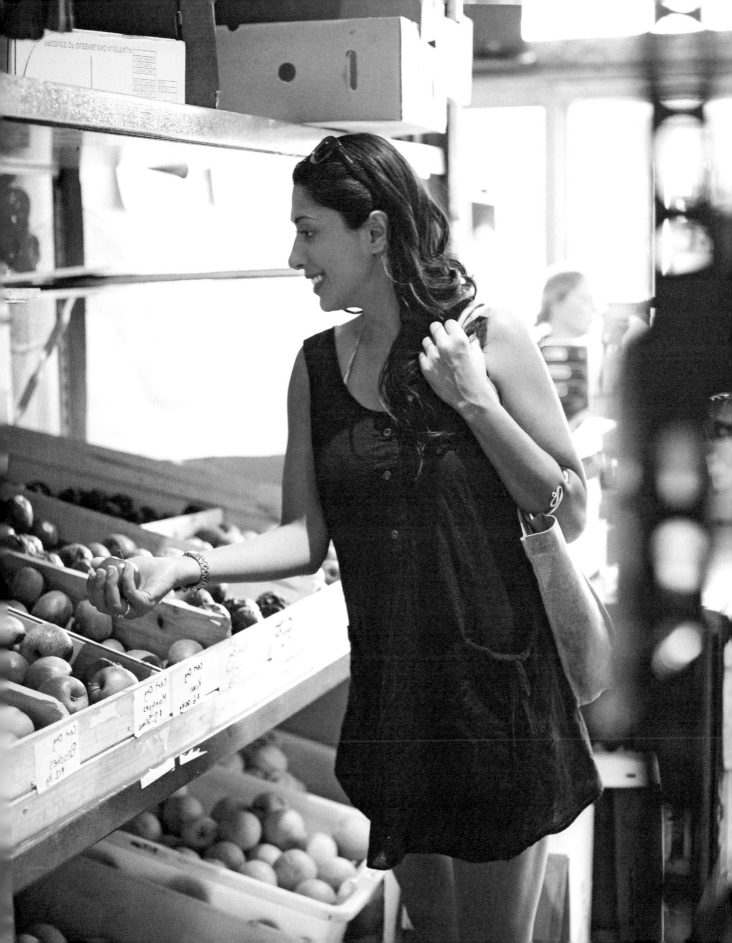

WEEK ONE: DETOXIFICATION PHASE

The art of a successful detox is in the planning – from preparing your mind by setting goals and clearing your work and social calendars as much as possible, to preparing your body by doing the shopping before you start, and clearing your pantry and fridge of the things you might crave during the detoxification phase. If you are someone who needs support, ask your family or friends if they'll do the program with you, or at least let them know you are doing it and ask them to help you if you feel tempted, or to support you emotionally if you need it. Remember also, you can get extra support by going to see a naturopath who can help you with everything from counselling, aiding you in letting go of your symptoms and emotions, right through to making up individualised herbal formulas and specialised supplement advice.

For optimum results, the Detoxification Phase should be followed for seven days. And remember, it is only a week out of your life – you might feel a little sorry for yourself and a little 'detoxy', but when it's finished, you'll experience abundant and true health, helping you achieve your best inside and out. What you really can look forward to is clear skin, bright eyes, lightness of being, a happy and positive mood, increased vitality and energy, clarity of mind, a stronger sense of who you are, and of course a slimmer body – all because you have taken the time to do this first week!

GENERAL TIPS

1. Wherever possible, try to source organic produce to limit chemical residue entering our bodies and our Earth.

2. Drink pure, high-quality water every day – this is vital for detoxification. Herbal tea does not count as part of your water intake. For increased alkalising effects, purchase a water ioniser.

3. Brush your skin daily on rising to detoxify your skin, improve your circulation and increase lymph flow. For type of brush and correct technique, see Detoxification Therapies in Guides and Tools, p 195.

4. Begin the day with an apple cider vinegar–cayenne shot (see p 140) to kick-start digestion and circulation.

5. Snacks (other than Go Green Juice (see p 142)) in mid-morning and mid-afternoon are optional. Try to eat only if you are hungry. *N.B. If weight loss is one of your goals and you're not succeeding, really try to avoid snacking, as well as eating after dinner. Instead, try having a cup of herbal tea or a glass of water with chlorophyll (this takes away sweet cravings too!).*

6. This is the strongest phase of the 14-day diet, where we will feel a little more tired and lacking energy, as our bodies go into detoxification mode. Therefore 20–30 minutes of gentle exercise each day is sufficient during this week, and if you can do some yoga at home, then this will be extremely beneficial. Even more important is being mindful about your breathing – take time to meditate or practise deep breathing or mindfulness exercises.

7. Enlist in some therapies too (see Guides and Tools on p 195) to help ease detoxification symptoms.

8. Keep an NET (nutrition, exercise, thought) diary (see Guides and Tools, p 199). This keeps track of everything you eat and drink, and just as importantly, of your thoughts, feelings and emotions. This helps you keep accountable and is also a great way to monitor your progress.

9. Choose three short-term goals (what you hope to achieve in the next two weeks); three medium-term goals (what you hope to achieve in the next three to six weeks); and three long-term goals (what you hope to achieve in the next three to six months). It is a very simple, powerful and affirming tool to revisit these goals on a daily basis (see Goal-setting in Part One: Movement, p 27).

GENTLE DETOX TIPS

- Drink 500 ml water four times daily – on rising, mid-morning, mid-afternoon and after dinner (finishing up at least one hour before bed). Make sure you drink at least twenty minutes away from your meals, so you don't disrupt your digestive juices.

- Always have one 250 ml glass of either Go Green Juice or a smoothie daily (include 1 tablespoon of chia seeds, flaxseed or LSA meal and 1 tablespoon of liquid essential fatty acids as explained in the recipe for Go Green Juice on p 142). The best time to drink Go Green Juice is first thing in the morning but any time before 4 p.m. is fine.

- Aim for one liquid main meal per day; try to make this soup for dinner. If you have to eat out, you can swap so you have soup for lunch and protein with salad or vegies for dinner, but only once this week.

If you have a sweet tooth, and really, really want to have something sweet after dinner, you may add 1 small teaspoon of organic raw honey to your tea or indulge in a maximum of two squares of raw cacao 'chocolate' (these tend to be made with coconut oil and agave syrup and include peppermint or other natural flavours). If you haven't had some plain, natural sheep milk or goat's milk yoghurt for the day, you may also have 1 tablespoon of sheep or goat's milk yoghurt with a drizzle of raw honey or agave syrup.

ADVANCED DETOX TIPS

For those of you who have done plenty of detoxes before and know what you're doing, you might want to try this advanced version of the Aussie Body Diet. The biggest difference in terms of food from the Gentle program is that during the Advanced Program's Detoxification Phase, you'll be avoiding all grains and all dairy.

During this week, aim for two liquid meals and one food-combined meal per day – Go Green Juice for breakfast and soup for dinner. If eating out, you can swap lunch and dinner, so you have soup for lunch and a food-combined meal at dinner.

You also have the option to include the Detox Drink, which is a strong detoxification enhancer. Detox Drink (see Liquids for all Phases, p 141 for recipe) is to be drunk 20 minutes before breakfast, lunch and dinner. This needs to be made up freshly, so if you are going to work or if you are out all day, take your supplements with you and mix them together at the appropriate times.

- Drink 750 ml water four times daily – on rising, mid-morning, mid-afternoon and after dinner (finishing up at least one hour before bed). Make sure you drink at least twenty minutes away from your meals, so you don't disrupt your digestive juices.

- Supplement your diet with Detox Drink three times daily. This is best taken 20 minutes before each meal.

- Substitute Go Green Juice for breakfast (300–350 ml glass and include 1 tablespoon of chia seeds, flaxseed or LSA meal and 1 tablespoon of liquid essential fatty acids). Aim to have only this until midday.

- Aim to have your main meal at lunch (midday) and try to make it a food-combined meal. Try to avoid all grains during this phase, so lunch will be protein and vegies.

- Aim to have your other liquid meal (soup) at dinner.

PORTION SIZE

Your stomach is actually not very big. If more than two fistful-sized amounts of food enter your stomach at once, it has a hell of a job to do. Its capacity to 'churn' the food (its normal process of mixing chewed food with gastric juices to complete digestion) is greatly burdened due to the excess inside it.

So eating less has more benefits than just looking great at the beach - it is in fact better for your digestion.

I'm not a believer in controlling portion size by counting calories or kilojoules or weighing food. Just stick to this simple rule and you can't go wrong:

One fist = snack size

Two fists = meal size

The palm of your hand = grain or meat quantity in any one sitting

DETOX REACTIONS

Detoxing can release toxins into the bloodstream, causing 'withdrawal' or detox symptoms, also known as a 'healing crisis'. This is part of the process – things get a little worse before they get better. These yucky symptoms are usually alleviated by Day 5 or 6, and you can look forward to abundant energy and a shining radiant self.

Remember you may have built up these toxins in your system over years. Don't expect to get rid of all of them in an afternoon. It can take a few weeks or even a number of programs spread throughout the year to get the result you want. Here is some advice on how to deal with detox reactions if they arise.

Headaches are common during a detox, especially if you are used to drinking caffeine. The pain can range from dull to throbbing, shooting, sharp or stabbing pain.

Recommendations:

- Drink plenty of water – hydrate, hydrate, hydrate.

- Ensure adequate amount of sleep (general recommendation eight hours a night).

- Magnesium relaxes arteries and muscles in the body and assists in reducing stress, anxiety, depression and insomnia.

Nausea – this can be due to lymph glands releasing toxins at such a fast rate that the liver has to manage the excess. It is then excreted, along with bile, into the stomach.

Recommendations:

- Water with fresh lemon juice and a pinch of salt.

- Ginger or peppermint tea.

Diarrhoea – can be a good sign unless it is excessive (over 4 times per day).

Recommendations:

- Fibre from whole grains, vegetables and psyllium husks helps to bulk the stool.

- Probiotics reduce inflammation and maintain health and integrity of the gastrointestinal tract.

Constipation – this is common, largely due to a sudden change in diet.

Recommendations:

- Increase your water intake.

- Try drinking a litre of warm water with 1 teaspoon of sea salt on rising.

- Castor oil is an age-old remedy to treat constipation – the dose will depend on the person. 1–2 tablespoons can be used in the evening, or in the morning before food. Follow with 1 cup of warm water. If 1 tablespoon does not work after three nights, increase to 2 tablespoons.

Mucus discharge – this is a common detox symptom as the lymphatic system expels mucus through the nose and throat.

Recommendations:

- Use a Neti Pot to help release discharge from sinuses.

- Add garlic to the diet to fight off infection and boost the immune system.

Body odour – due to toxins being released from lymph nodes and pores under armpit.

Recommendations:

- Use natural, pH-balanced soaps and skincare products to maintain your skin. Try bathing in an apple cider vinegar wash twice a week – pour two cups of apple cider vinegar in your bath.

Spirulina or chlorophyll are natural deodorisers which reduce body odour and bad breath. Alfalfa and parsley are both excellent sources of chlorophyll.

Rashes and pimples – as the skin is one of our largest elimination systems, skin problems are common as toxins are released.

Recommendations:

- Increase your water intake, starting with a cup of warm to hot water upon rising

- Zinc helps to repair damaged tissues, heal wounds and reduce inflammation

- Tea tree oil applied topically to pimples to dry them out

Coated tongue – normal during a cleanse due to accumulated toxins being released.

Recommendations:

- Brush your tongue with a toothbrush or better yet, use a tongue scraper.

Dizziness/light-headedness – this can happen when you make a radical change to your diet.

Recommendations:

- Increase water intake and add electrolytes

- Coconut water

- Add a spoonful of raw honey to a glass of warm water or herbal tea

Fatigue – as you are eating less, it is common to feel fatigued, especially if you are used to eating a lot. This is temporary and once you have completed your detox, your energy levels will increase.

Recommendations:

- Avoid excess exercise: gentle exercise is helpful during a detox but don't overdo it.

- Have early nights and give your body adequate rest.

Muscle cramping/aches/pains – this can indicate the redistribution of toxins into the connective tissue as the body tries to flush them out.

Recommendations:

- Add electrolytes to your water as your body needs salt and magnesium, or drink coconut water

- Massage and/or gentle stretching and yoga

- Saunas and Epsom salt baths can also help relieve aches and pains

Excessive gas/flatulence – this is common with a sudden change in diet.

Recommendations:

- Fenugreek seeds soaked in water overnight and drunk first thing in the morning are very effective in reducing gas

- Fennel tea

Bloating – another gastrointestinal symptom common due to a sudden change in diet.

Recommendations:

- Ginger or peppermint tea

- Probiotics

- Exercise to relieve bloating: lie flat on your back and bring your left knee to your chest while keeping your right leg as close to the floor as possible. Hug your left knee to the count of 20. Release and repeat with your right knee. Alternate knees five times or more, depending on the severity of symptoms.

Frequent urination – this is common as you are taking in a lot of fluids to flush unwanted toxins out of your body. Urination frequency will become normal when your detox is complete.

DAVID THOMPSON, *chef and author*

It was time. Nothing was really the matter, but having turned fifty I realised that if I wanted to stay fit, trim and spry I needed to look after myself – to change a few things. One of my friends had hands gnarled with arthritis but within a few months of detoxing and dieting, they were freed from its stony grip. Such a remarkable transformation convinced me that I should do the same. And this was the way I met Saimaa.

A chatty consultation lead to the inevitable imposition of a diet: no dairy products, no booze, no wheat or fermented products and no coffee: hard choices for a six-espresso-a-day man who finished the day with a decent glass of pinot noir. Mostly, though, the diet was quite liberal: a little organic meat, some fish, some grains – though no wheat or white rice – and bundles of fruits and vegetables. This along with a programme of dietary supplements, pills and colonic irrigation would help to disgorge the sins of my past.

It was too easy, too liberal, really. So I decided to undertake a much stricter regime: one of mostly raw vegetables combined with small humane doses of contrabands. I was quite firm and stuck to this for four weeks. I also worked out at the gym, an hour or so each morning, six days a week. I was on a determined mission.

My God, things changed quickly. I became energetic and enthusiastic with a feeling of general wellbeing and lightness, both emotionally and physically. More than that, I felt rejuvenated, with unreasonable amounts of optimism, and happiness. My short-term memory, which had been lagging, returned to the acuity of my thirties.

When I ate I was very aware of what I was eating. I didn't overeat but I wasn't dissatisfied. I rarely felt bloated or heavy. Every morning I woke up with a clear mind. It was easier to maintain than I thought because the palpable benefits of the diet far outweighed any longing for other delicious but illicit food.

I am off the more stringent parts of the diet now. Although I am very aware of what I eat, making sure that most of the diet is healthy, consisting mostly of vegetables and fruit. There are times when I fall back into eating chocolate, crunchy bread, cheese and charcuterie but they are occasional pleasures without dire effects. Even when I have a night with my old friend pinot noir, the next day is still clear, unburdened with the cloudiness of the past.

This detoxing and dieting has cleansed my system and has made me feel refreshed and resilient. I travel the globe a few times a year and have to confirm that Saimaa's program, health spa, support and service are second to none.

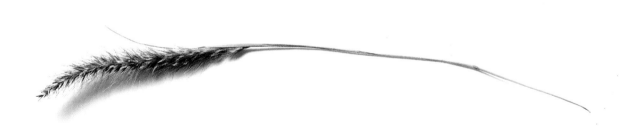

DETOXIFICATION PHASE RECIPES

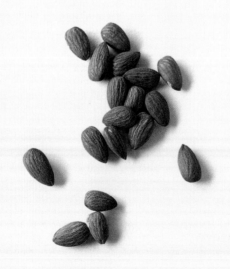

BREAKFAST

Ancient Grain Porridge 56
Delicious Muesli 56
Organic Egg & Zucchini Pancakes 58
Buckwheat Pancakes 58

LUNCH

Stuffed Capsicums 60
Salmon Salad with Asparagus & Roast Tomato 60
Fish with Fresh Tomato Salsa 62
Ladakhi Chicken Curry 64
Zucchini 'Pasta' with Creamy Sauce 64

SOUPS & BROTHS

Vegetable Stock 66
Fragrant Soup 66
Energy Soup.. 68
Zucchini & Coriander Soup 68
Spinach & Seaweed Soup.. 69
Simple Avocado Soup... 69
Spicy Pumpkin Soup.. 70
Creamy Herb & Cucumber Soup............................... 70

BREAKFAST

ANCIENT GRAIN PORRIDGE

A warming gluten-free porridge that is easy to prepare and very filling and nourishing to eat.

SERVES 2

250 ml water
250 ml almond or rice milk
2 tablespoons amaranth flakes
2 tablespoons quinoa flakes
1 ripe medium pear, coarsely grated
2 tablespoons chia seeds, soaked overnight
2 teaspoons raw honey or agave syrup
ground cinnamon

Heat water and milk nearly to a simmer over a medium heat in a small saucepan. Add amaranth and quinoa flakes along with pear.

Cook for 3–4 minutes, stirring often, until porridge reaches a thick consistency.

Serve in bowls with chia seeds and honey drizzled over the top, and a sprinkle of cinnamon.

DELICIOUS MUESLI >

This gluten-free muesli can be eaten straight away with a sliced banana for extra sweetness and/or two tablespoons of sheep's milk, goat's milk or natural yoghurt. Or it can be kept in the fridge for three to four days in an airtight container. You can vary the taste simply by changing the milk – during the detoxification phase, you can use quinoa, nut or seed milk.

SERVES 4

20 g puffed quinoa
20 g puffed amaranth
40 g rice bran
30 g pepitas
30 g shredded coconut
30 g chia seeds
30 g dates
30 g goji berries (or any type of berries)
250 ml rice milk
yoghurt, to serve (optional)
sliced bananas or berries, to serve (optional)

Place all ingredients in a bowl and mix well to combine. Add yoghurt and/or sliced bananas or berries for taste.

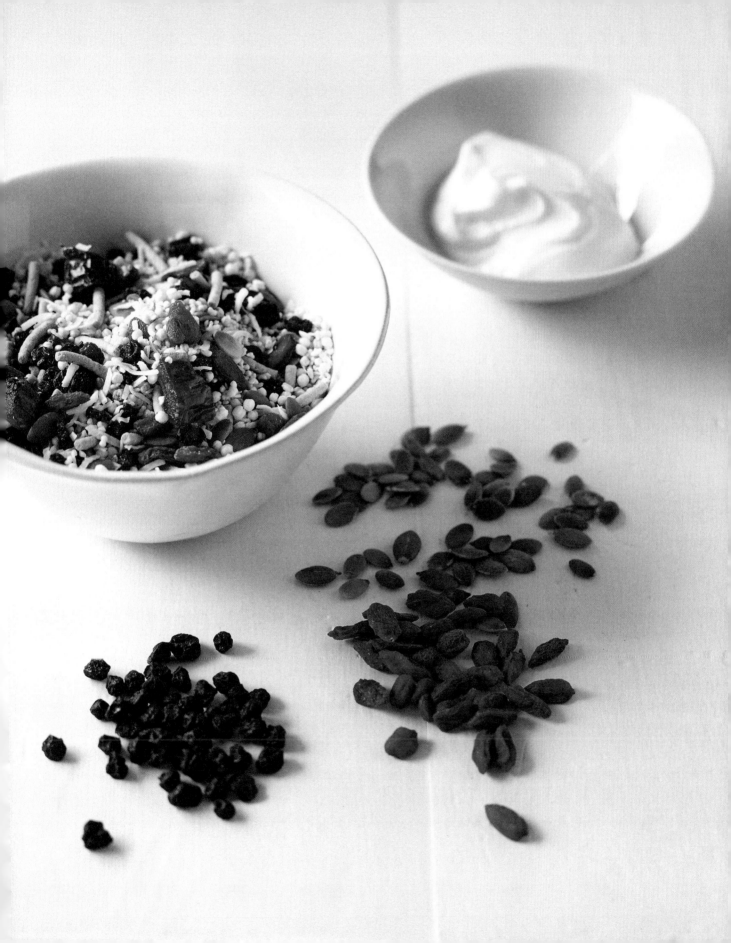

ORGANIC EGG & ZUCCHINI PANCAKES

A protein-rich meal that's incredibly easy to prepare. During the detoxification phase, please try to only consume organic, free-range eggs to reduce the level of toxin exposure. Serve with a squeeze of lemon juice, and perhaps with a side of wilted spinach and fresh tomato.

SERVES 1

2 eggs
1 medium zucchini (courgette) (120 g), grated
olive oil, for frying
sea salt and freshly ground black pepper

Whisk the eggs in a small bowl until thoroughly combined, add grated zucchini, and combine with salt and pepper to taste.

Heat a little oil in a frying pan over medium heat, drop 3–4 tablespoons of the mixture into the pan and cook for 1 minute or so until golden brown, then flip and cook on the other side for about 1 minute. Repeat with the rest of the mixture.

BUCKWHEAT PANCAKES >

For this recipe, you do need a blender or food processor to break up the coconut into the desired consistency. If you don't have one, you can substitute coconut cream. These pancakes are very versatile and can be served sweet or savoury – try sheep's yoghurt, fresh fruit and almond butter, or avocado, wilted spinach and cherry tomatoes.

SERVES 2

1 medium young coconut
80 g buckwheat flour
30 g flaxseed
1 teaspoon coconut butter, melted
pinch sea salt or Himalayan rock salt
2 tablespoons (30 g) pumpkin seeds
2 tablespoons (30 g) sunflower seeds
olive oil, for frying

Blend 175 g of the flesh and 250 ml of the juice of the coconut until smooth.

Mix all ingredients except pumpkin and sunflower seeds in a large mixing bowl until you have a smooth batter. The mixture should be quite gelatinous and sticky.

Mix pumpkin seeds and sunflower seeds together in a small bowl. Scoop out 1½ tablespoons of mix and set aside in a small bowl. Add remainder of seed mix to buckwheat batter and mix together.

Heat a little olive oil in a frying pan over medium heat and drop about 3–4 tablespoons of batter into the pan. Cook for 1 minute and then sprinkle a teaspoon of the seed mix on top. Cook for another 30 seconds and then flip the pancake over. Cook for a further 2–3 minutes until pancake is golden brown and repeat with the rest of the mixture.

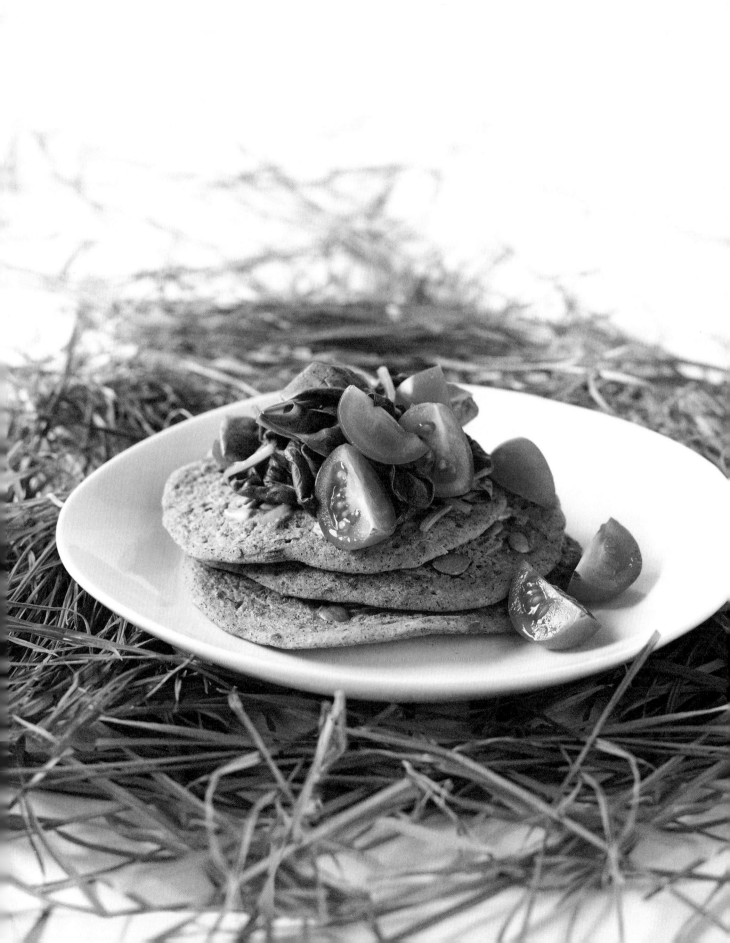

LUNCH

STUFFED CAPSICUMS

A popular vegan dish. Add goat's cheese on top for extra protein and flavour during the detoxification phase.

SERVES 6

3 small red capsicums (peppers)
2 medium zucchini (courgettes), finely diced
4 green onions (320 g), thinly sliced
100 g green beans, trimmed and sliced into
    5 cm lengths
1 × 300 g tin cannellini beans, rinsed and drained
1 tablespoon olive oil
2 tablespoons pine nuts

SAUCE

1 × 800 g tin crushed tomato
2 cloves garlic, minced
1 tablespoon raw apple cider vinegar
sea salt and freshly ground black pepper
big handful of fresh basil leaves, torn

Preheat oven to 200°C.

Halve capsicums lengthways, scoop out seeds and trim membranes, then place cut-side-up in a large baking dish.

To make sauce, heat all ingredients except basil in a saucepan over medium heat, bring to a simmer, then reduce for 15 minutes while you prepare the filling. Stir through most of the basil, reserving some.

Combine zucchini, onion, green beans, cannellini beans and olive oil, spoon into capsicum halves, top with sauce and sprinkle over pine nuts.

Bake for 30 minutes until tender and serve sprinkled with remaining basil.

SALMON SALAD WITH ASPARAGUS & ROAST TOMATO

A wonderful combination of salmon and egg makes this yummy salad high in essential fatty acids and complete in amino acids.

SERVES 2

2 salmon fillets (440 g), skin removed
    and pin-boned
250 g cherry tomatoes, halved
2 tablespoons olive oil
170 g asparagus, trimmed and cut into 5 cm lengths
50 g baby rocket leaves
juice of ½ lemon
1 tablespoon raw apple cider vinegar
1 tablespoon flaxseed oil
2 eggs, soft boiled, shelled and quartered
sea salt and freshly ground black pepper

Preheat oven to 200°C.

Place cherry tomatoes, cut side up, on a baking tray. Drizzle tomatoes with olive oil and bake for 12–15 minutes. Set aside to cool.

Plunge asparagus into a saucepan of boiling salted water for a minute to blanch, then run under cold water and drain.

Grill or chargrill salmon for 4 minutes. Coarsely flake salmon, combine in a bowl with tomatoes, asparagus and rocket. Whisk together lemon juice, vinegar and flaxseed oil for the dressing. Serve salad in bowls with a drizzle of dressing and top each with egg, then season with salt and pepper to taste.

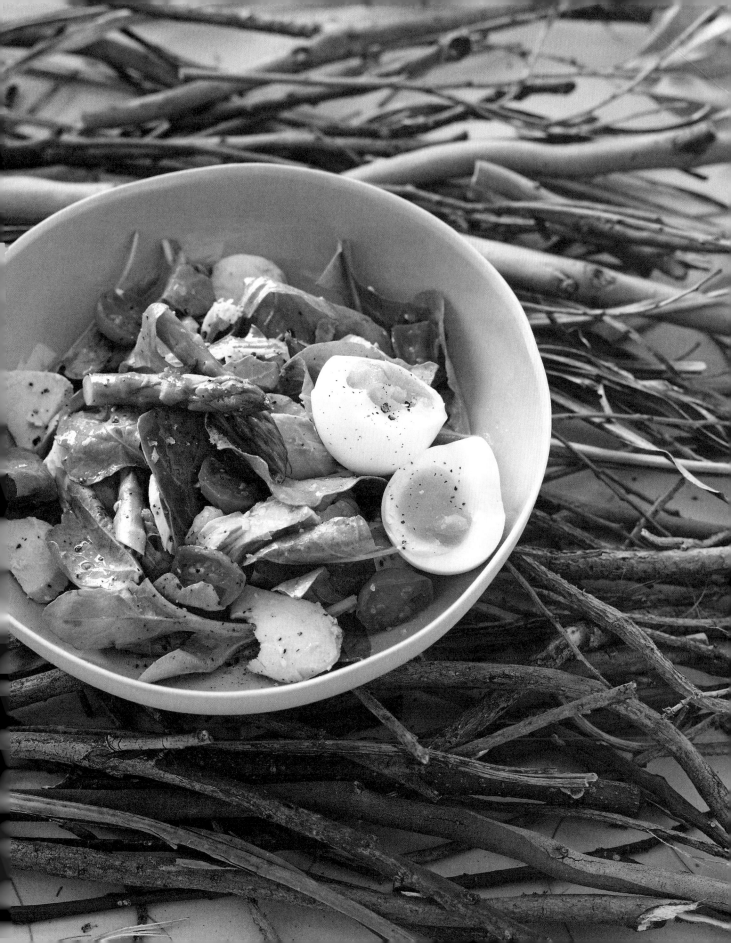

FISH WITH FRESH TOMATO SALSA

I have suggested using blue-eye trevalla in this recipe and during the Detoxification Phase, but it is delicious with all kinds of white fish. You can chargrill instead of pan-frying if you prefer.

SERVES 4

3 tomatoes (450 g), finely chopped or 450 g mixed cherry tomatoes, quartered

1 medium red capsicum (pepper) (200 g), seeded and finely chopped

½ cup finely chopped basil or flat-leaf parsley

½ medium red onion (170 g), finely chopped

2 teaspoons dried oregano

1 fresh red chilli, seeded and finely minced

1 clove garlic, minced

2 tablespoons raw apple cider vinegar

60 ml olive oil

sea salt and freshly ground black pepper

4 × 185 g blue-eye trevalla fillets

200 g mixed salad leaves

Combine tomato, capsicum, herbs and onion in a bowl with chilli, garlic, oregano, vinegar and olive oil. Season with salt and pepper and set aside.

Pan-fry or barbecue fish fillets for 3–4 minutes each side, until just cooked.

Serve fish with salsa and mixed salad leaves.

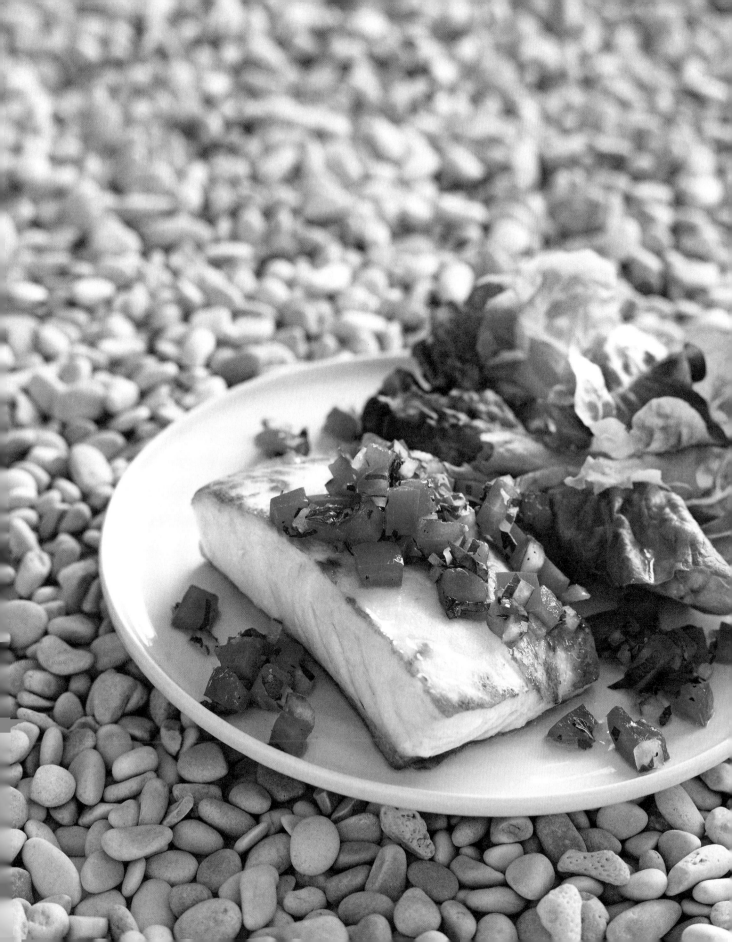

LADAKHI CHICKEN CURRY

This simple but deliciously fragrant chicken curry was provided by Christine Manfield, chef, author and champion detoxer. It comes from her book *Tasting India* and the recipe originates from the Indian region of Ladakh.

SERVES 4

2 red onions, roughly chopped
8 cloves garlic, roughly chopped
1 tablespoon roughly chopped ginger
2 fresh green chillies, roughly chopped
3 ripe tomatoes, roughly chopped
1 teaspoon chilli powder
2 tablespoons vegetable oil
800 g organic chicken breast fillets, sliced into thin strips
2 teaspoons sea salt
2 tablespoons chopped coriander leaves
steamed rice or vegies, to serve

Put onion, garlic, ginger, chilli, tomato and chilli powder into a food processor and blend until smooth.

Heat oil in a frying pan and add chicken. Fry over medium heat for 1 minute only, then remove from pan and set aside.

Tip onion and tomato paste into the same pan and fry over medium heat for 40 minutes until softened and sauce-like, adding a little water if it appears too dry.

Add chicken and stir into sauce until well coated. Cook for 3 minutes or until cooked through, then season with salt and remove from the heat. Stir through fresh coriander and serve hot with steamed rice.

ZUCCHINI 'PASTA' WITH CREAMY SAUCE

An amazingly filling dish which will make normal pasta feel too heavy! Garnish with crumbled goat's cheese for extra protein.

SERVES 4

4 large zucchini (courgettes) (600 g)
2 tablespoons olive oil
¼ cup basil leaves, torn and a few whole leaves reserved

SAUCE

150 g macadamias
15 g sun-dried tomatoes
juice of ½ lemon
2 cloves garlic, minced
1 teaspoon sea salt
freshly ground black pepper

To make the sauce, place macadamia nuts and sun-dried tomatoes in separate bowls, cover each with water and leave to soak for 30 minutes.

Using a potato peeler, peel zucchini into long strips, then slice strips lengthways to create 'spaghetti'. Place in a large bowl, combine with olive oil and sliced basil and set aside.

Drain macadamia nuts and sun-dried tomatoes (reserving the water you soaked the tomatoes in) and place in food processor along with lemon juice, garlic, salt and pepper. Pulse to combine, then with the motor running slowly add reserved tomato water and blend until the mixture forms a creamy consistency.

Stir sauce through zucchini 'pasta' until well combined, garnish with a few whole basil leaves and serve.

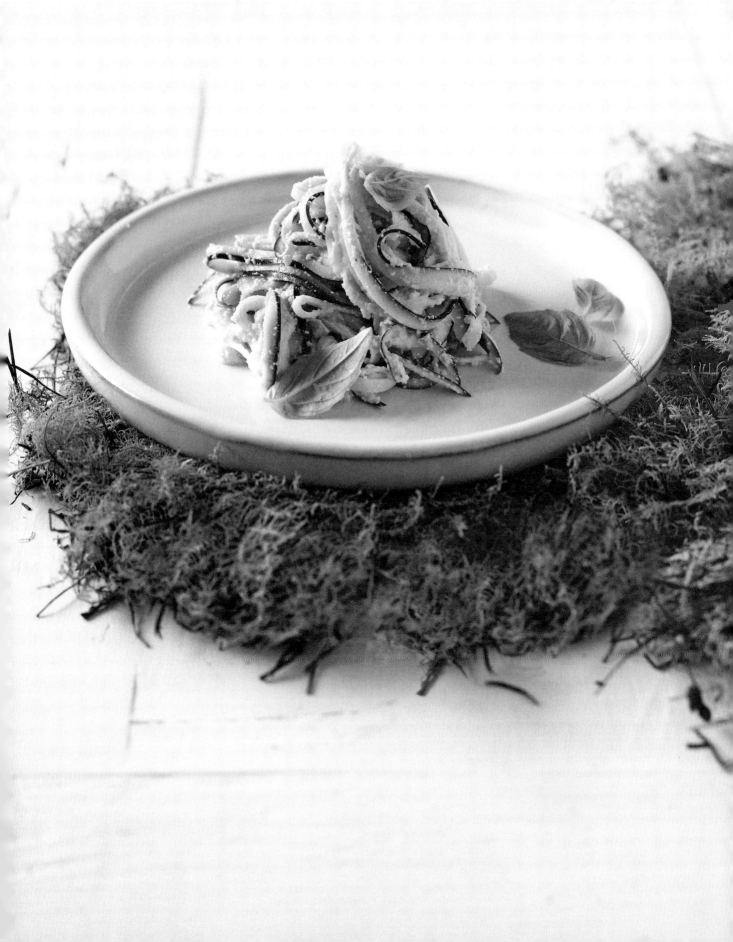

SOUPS & BROTHS

VEGETABLE STOCK

This stock can be used as a basis for the Fragrant Soup opposite, to flavour casseroles and stews. It can also be enjoyed on its own by leaving the vegetables in. This stock will keep for 3 days in the fridge, or up to 3 months in the freezer.

MAKES 1.5 LITRES

1 tablespoon olive oil
2 onions (300 g), finely chopped
3 cloves garlic, minced
2 carrots (240 g), roughly chopped
2 stalks celery (200 g), roughly chopped
1 turnip (230 g), roughly chopped
1 parsnip (250 g), roughly chopped
2 bay leaves
6 black peppercorns
3 teaspoons miso paste
sea salt and freshly ground black pepper

Heat olive oil in a large saucepan over medium heat, add onion and garlic and cook for 2 minutes until soft. Add remaining vegetables and cook, covered, for 10 minutes, shaking the pan often.

Cover vegetables with 3 litres water, bring to the boil and add bay leaves and peppercorns. Simmer, covered, for 1½ hours, then turn off the heat, strain out the vegetables and stir through the miso paste. Add salt and pepper to taste.

FRAGRANT SOUP >

The crisp yet tender vegetables floating in a delicate turmeric-infused broth make this a very attractive, light yet filling dish.

SERVES 2

1 carrot (120 g), diced
45 g broccoli, cut into florets
50 g cauliflower, cut into florets
85 g asparagus, cut into 5 cm lengths
1 golden shallot (40 g), peeled and left whole
500 ml boiling water
500 ml iced water
600 ml vegetable stock (see opposite)
5 cm piece galangal (25 g), roughly chopped
1 lemongrass stalk, roughly chopped
1 fresh red chilli
5 cm piece fresh turmeric root (25 g),
    roughly chopped
2 tablespoons coriander leaves, plus extra to serve
2 kaffir lime leaves

Place carrot, broccoli, cauliflower, asparagus and shallot in a saucepan with the boiling water then blanch for about 15 seconds, then drain and plunge into a bowl of iced water.

Heat vegetable stock in a saucepan until it begins to simmer. Put galangal, lemongrass, chilli, turmeric, coriander and kaffir lime leaves into a tea infuser or muslin bag, drop into stock and simmer for 2 minutes.

Add blanched vegetables to soup, and allow to heat through for 30 seconds. Remove tea infuser or bag with spices and discard.

Serve garnished with extra coriander leaves.

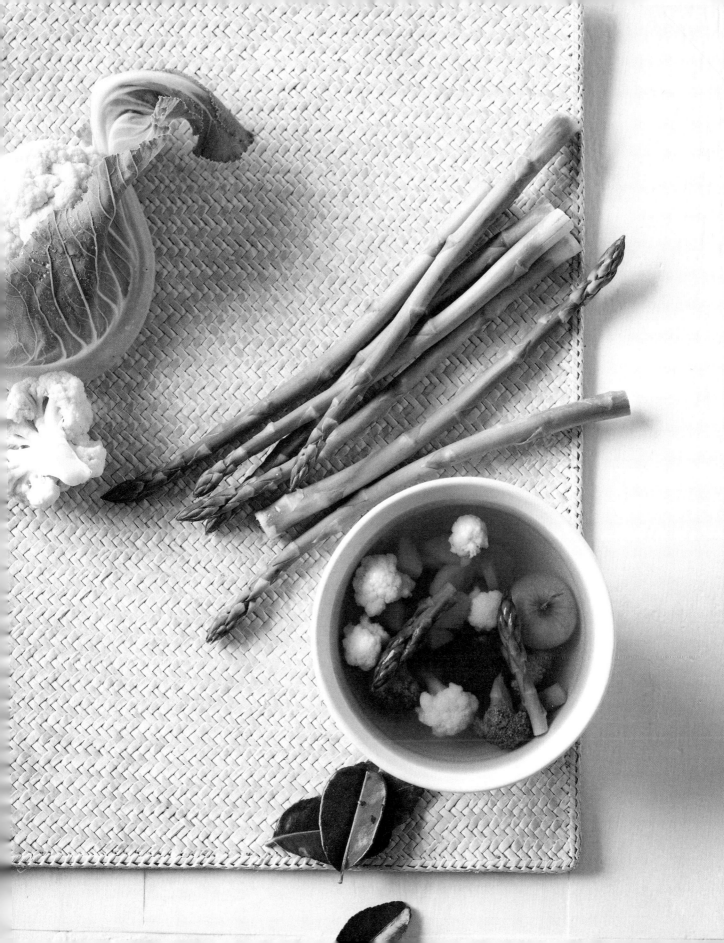

ENERGY SOUP

This recipe contains dulse, a sea vegetable that is packed with vitamins and minerals. You can buy it as flakes or in larger pieces. Energy Soup works well with a variety of toppings, such as diced avocado, minced garlic, soaked sun-dried tomatoes, sliced spring onions, diced capsicum (pepper) or spirulina powder.

SERVES 2

juice of 1 lemon
125 ml cold-pressed olive or flaxseed oil
50 g dulse or dulse flakes
1 raw nori sheet, torn into smaller pieces
2 medium tomatoes (300 g), quartered
125 g spinach leaves, washed and roughly chopped
2 stalks celery (200 g), roughly chopped
1 medium green cucumber (170 g), peeled and
    roughly chopped
1½ cups fresh basil or coriander leaves
    (or a mix of both)
40 g raw hemp seeds or raw pine nuts (80 g)
1 teaspoon sea salt or Himalayan salt
½ teaspoon chilli or cayenne powder, to taste

Put all ingredients in blender, then process on high speed with a cup of filtered water and puree until creamy. Serve in bowls with your choice of toppings.

ZUCCHINI & CORIANDER SOUP

A premium detox soup due to the large quantity of coriander, known for its ability to remove heavy metals from the body.

SERVES 2

1 zucchini (120 g), diced
1 carrot (120 g), diced
1 stalk celery (150 g)
¼ red onion (60 g), finely chopped
1 tablespoon flaxseed oil
80 g coriander leaves, torn, plus a few
    extra finely shredded for garnish
½ teaspoon sea salt
¼ medium avocado (30 g)
freshly ground black pepper

Blend all ingredients together with 4 cups of filtered water on high speed until smooth. Heat in a saucepan until warm, garnish with fresh coriander and serve.

SPINACH & SEAWEED SOUP

A wonderfully tasty soup, packed with powerhouse nutrients and essential fatty acids derived from the different seaweeds.

SERVES 2

1 zucchini (courgette) (120 g), diced
1 carrot (120 g), diced
1 stalk celery (100 g), roughly chopped
1 leek (350 g), trimmed and roughly chopped
1 tablespoon flaxseed oil, plus extra for drizzling
¼ medium avocado (65 g)
125 g spinach leaves, washed and roughly chopped
2 tablespoons kelp powder
sea salt
1 tablespoon dulse flakes

Blend all ingredients except salt and dulse together with 4 cups filtered water in a blender for 3 minutes or until smooth.

Season and serve garnished with dulse and a drizzle of olive oil.

SIMPLE AVOCADO SOUP

Adjust the amount of jalapeno chilli you use in this recipe according to how much heat you enjoy. Serve garnished with bean sprouts or coriander.

SERVES 2

2 medium avocados (500 g), cut into 1 cm dice
½–1 jalapeno chilli, seeds removed and finely chopped
1 teaspoon ground coriander
1 teaspoon wheat-free tamari
¼ teaspoon freshly ground black pepper
½ teaspoon sea salt or Himalayan rock salt
flesh of 1 lime, diced
coriander leaves, to garnish

Combine all ingredients except lime and coriander in a bowl, then put half the mixture in the blender and blend until smooth.

Pour blended mixture back into the bowl and fold in to combine with unblended mixture.

Add 125 ml water if you want a thinner texture.

SPICY PUMPKIN SOUP

It may seem unusual, but the pumpkin and other vegetables are left raw in this recipe to preserve all the nutrients. I have suggested parsley for the garnish here, but you can use any herb you prefer.

SERVES 2

500 g butternut pumpkin, peeled and diced
4 carrots (480 g), diced
1 red capsicum (pepper) (150 g), seeded and diced
½ red onion (170 g), finely chopped
1 clove garlic, minced
½ stalk celery (50 g), finely sliced
2 tablespoons flaxseed oil, plus extra for drizzling
1½ tablespoons raw apple cider vinegar
1 teaspoon wheat-free tamari
1 teaspoon sea salt
juice of 5 cm piece of ginger (25 g), passed
    through a juicer
pinch cayenne pepper
chopped flat-leaf parsley, to garnish

Blend all ingredients except parsley together with 1 litre filtered water on high speed for about 3 minutes, or until smooth.

Serve either slightly warm or at room temperature with parsley.

CREAMY HERB & CUCUMBER SOUP >

A refreshing soup, especially for the warmer months. Best served chilled.

SERVES 2

3 green cucumbers (500 g), peeled and seeded
1 lemon (140 g), peeled, cut into chunks and
    seeded
200 g natural sheep's yoghurt
1 clove garlic, minced
40 g crushed walnuts
1 teaspoon flaxseed oil
¼ cup flat-leaf parsley, chopped
¼ cup mint leaves, chopped
chopped fresh chives, to garnish (optional)

Blend everything except mint and chives together with 1 litre water in a high-speed blender for 3 minutes or until smooth. Add mint and blend for a further 15 seconds, then chill for 1 hour and serve with chives if desired.

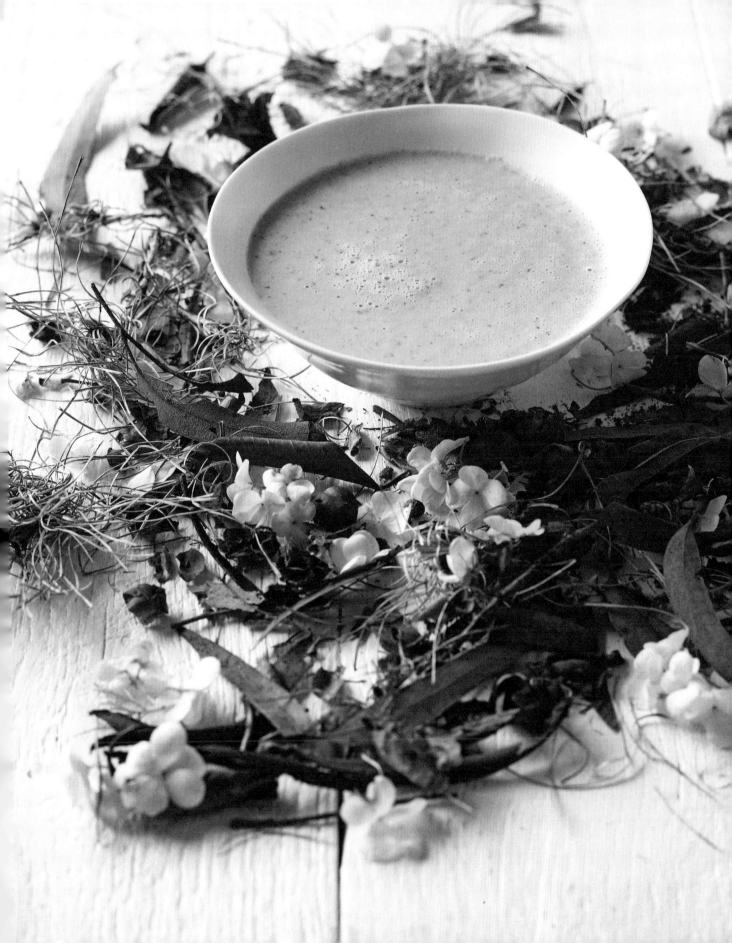

DETOX PHASE MENU PLANNER – GENTLE CHART

	MONDAY	TUESDAY	WEDNESDAY	THURSDAY	FRIDAY	SATURDAY	SUNDAY
On rising	500 ml water Apple cider vinegar–cayenne shot	500 ml water Apple cider vinegar–cayenne shot	500 ml water Apple cider vinegar–cayenne shot	500 ml water Apple cider vinegar–cayenne shot	500 ml water Apple cider vinegar–cayenne shot	500 ml water Apple cider vinegar–cayenne shot	500 ml water Apple cider vinegar–cayenne shot
Breakfast	Delicious Muesli Herbal tea	Sun Salute Smoothie Herbal tea	Ancient Grain Porridge Herbal tea	Organic Egg and Zucchini Pancakes Herbal tea	Delicious Muesli Herbal tea	Downward Dog Smoothie Herbal tea	Buckwheat Pancakes Herbal tea
Mid-morning	250 ml Go Green Juice 500 ml water	250 ml Go Green Juice 500 ml water	250 ml Go Green Juice 500 ml water	250 ml Go Green Juice 500 ml water	250 ml Go Green Juice 500 ml water	250 ml Go Green Juice 500 ml water	250 ml Go Green Juice 500 ml water
Lunch	Stuffed Capsicums	Salmon Salad with Asparagus & Roast Tomato	Ladakhi Chicken Curry	Salmon & Zucchini Frittata	Zucchini Pasta with Creamy Sauce	Chicken Cacciatore	Fish with Fresh Tomato Salsa
Snacks (only if needed)	500 ml water Handful mixed nuts	500 ml water Crudites with avocado dip	500 ml water Brown rice cakes with tahini	500 ml water Piece of fruit	500 ml water Crudites with hummus	500 ml water Rice crackers with avocado	500 ml water 2 tbsps kefir or natural yoghurt
Dinner	Fragrant Soup 500 ml water	Energy Soup 500 ml water	Creamy Herb & Cucumber Soup 500 ml water	Spinach & Seaweed Soup 500 ml water	Simple Avocado Soup 500 ml water	Warm Zucchini & Coriander Soup 500 ml water	Spicy Pumpkin Soup 500 ml water
After dinner (optional, only if needed)	1 cup ginger, lemon and honey tea	1 cup peppermint tea with 1 teaspoon raw honey	2 squares raw cacao chocolate	2 tbsps kefir or natural yoghurt	1 cup peppermint tea with 1 tsp raw honey	1 cup ginger, lemon and honey tea	2 squares raw cacao chocolate

DETOX PHASE MENU PLANNER – **ADVANCED CHART**

	MONDAY	TUESDAY	WEDNESDAY	THURSDAY	FRIDAY	SATURDAY	SUNDAY
On rising	750 ml water Apple cider vinegar–cayenne shot	750 ml water Apple cider vinegar–cayenne shot	750 ml water Apple cider vinegar–cayenne shot	750 ml water Apple cider vinegar–cayenne shot	750 ml water Apple cider vinegar–cayenne shot	750 ml water Apple cider vinegar–cayenne shot	750 ml water Apple cider vinegar–cayenne shot
Breakfast	Detox drink 300–350 ml Go Green Juice	Detox drink 300–350 ml Go Green Juice	Detox drink 300–350 ml Go Green Juice	Detox drink 300–350 ml Go Green Juice	Detox drink 300–350 ml Go Green Juice	Detox drink 300–350 ml Go Green Juice	Detox drink 300–350 ml Go Green Juice
Mid-morning	750 ml water	750 ml water	750 ml water	750 ml water	750 ml water	750 ml water	750 ml water
Lunch	Detox drink Stuffed Capsicums	Detox drink Salmon Salad with Asparagus & Roast Tomato	Detox drink Ladakhi Chicken Curry (with vegies)	Detox drink Salmon & Zucchini Frittata	Detox drink Zucchini Pasta with Creamy Sauce	Detox drink Organic Egg and Zucchini Pancakes	Detox drink Fish with Fresh Tomato Salsa
Mid-afternoon	750 ml water	750 ml water	750 ml water	750 ml water	750 ml water	750 ml water	750 ml water
Dinner	Detox drink Fragrant Soup 750 ml water	Detox drink Energy Soup 750 ml water	Detox drink Creamy Herb & Cucumber Soup 750 ml water	Detox drink Spinach & Seaweed Soup 750 ml water	Detox drink Simple Avocado Soup 750 ml water	Detox drink Warm Zucchini & Coriander Soup 750 ml water	Detox drink Spicy Pumpkin Soup 750 ml water

N.B. Go Green Juice can be drunk either at mid-morning or mid-afternoon

WEEK TWO: NUTRITIVE PHASE

Congratulations – you've already completed the hardest part – it wasn't that difficult, was it? And now you have the added benefit of working within a clean canvas – your body will naturally want to eat less, will naturally crave alkalising foods in their whole forms, and you don't have to worry about counting calories or portion control. This is all because you have taken the time to detox, re-igniting your body's instincts about correct nutrition. Your body is already responding with gratitude – your muscular aches might be disappearing or have gone completely, your skin probably looks clearer, you have more vitality, you feel calmer, happier, and enjoy getting out of bed in the mornings.

Before going into Week 2, it's a great time to check in with your goals if you haven't done so already, and see for yourself how far you've come. Re-do your list of symptoms – think again about the ailments that have been affecting your health, and check to see whether they are disappearing, or have gone altogether.

The Nutritive Phase of the program is like sowing seeds in your garden after you've taken the weeds out. You can add more foods and observe that you don't put on weight; in fact you are probably still losing weight (because you've cleared your channels of elimination and increased the efficiency of your metabolism). Moreover, you can see how each type of food makes you feel, as your body is now clean and able to show you signs of distress more effectively.

This is also the week where you can start to increase movement, as naturally you will have much more energy, and you've re-ignited your mind and are therefore more disciplined and motivated to do so. But remember, your body is still repairing, so allow yourself to have time to reflect and contemplate, and slow down and rest when you need to.

GENERAL TIPS

1. Points 1 to 5 in General Detoxification Phase Tips on p 49 apply here.

2. Increase exercise to at least 45 minutes to 1 hour, five times this week. Include at least one yoga session.

3. Keep an NET diary (see Guides and Tools on p 199) to keep you on track and to monitor your progress.

4. Check in with your goals and use your weekly planner to monitor your progress.

5. Remember to breathe deeply, use therapies (see p 195) as aids, and spend time in sunshine and nature for their nutritive qualities.

GENTLE PROGRAM TIPS

- All whole grains except wheat are allowed during Nutritive Phase. You can start to re-introduce rye, spelt, oats and barley if you wish. Still no corn.

- Limit red meat to only organic lamb, which you can have up to three times per week. You can still have fish or organic chicken and turkey.

- You may alternate lunch and dinner if you wish, but aim for one liquid meal and one food-combined meal per day (see the Nutritive Phase Example Menu Planner on p 98).

ADVANCED TIPS

Follow the same guidelines as set out above, but aim to stick to gluten-free grains this week and keep avoiding all dairy.

During this week, aim for one liquid meal per day, and two food-combined meals per day. You also have the option to include the Algae Drink, which is a wonderful nutritive enhancer. Algae Drink (see p 140 for recipe) is to be drunk 20 minutes before breakfast, lunch and dinner. It needs to be made up fresh, so if you are going to work or if you are out all day, take the supplements with you in a container or sandwich bag, and mix it together at the appropriate times.

The most nutrient-dense foods on the planet are micro-algae. They are a potent source of antioxidants, carotenoids, vitamins, minerals, amino acids, polysaccharides, essential fatty acids, chlorophyll and phytonutrients – in a word, they are superfoods for you to fertilise your internal 'garden' with. Micro-algae include spirulina and marine phytoplankton (*Dunaliella salina*).

- Drink 750 ml water four times daily – on rising, mid-morning, mid-afternoon and after dinner (finishing up at least one hour before bed). Make sure you drink at least 20 minutes away from your meals, so you don't disrupt your digestive juices.

- Supplement with Algae Drink three times daily. This is best taken 20 minutes before breakfast, lunch and dinner.

- Substitute Go Green Juice for breakfast (300–350 ml glass and include 1 tablespoon of seeds or meal and 1 tablespoon liquid essential fatty acids). Aim to have only this till midday.

- Aim to have your main meal at lunch (midday) and try to make it a food-combined meal.

NUTRITIVE PHASE RECIPES

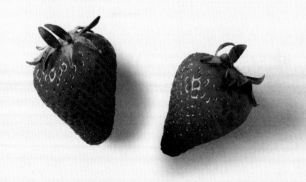

BREAKFAST

LUNCH

DINNER

SOUPS & BROTHS

BREAKFAST

EASY BIRCHER MUESLI

A delicious bircher muesli that's easy to put together – you just combine the ingredients and leave them to soak in the fridge overnight. Serve with natural yoghurt or an extra splash of milk.

SERVES 2

45 g rolled oats
2 tablespoons oat bran
1 tablespoon sunflower seeds
1 tablespoon chia seeds
1 tablespoon raw apple cider vinegar
70 g mixed berries such as goji, acai or blueberries
1 small banana (75 g)
1 tablespoon (20 g) shredded coconut
1 tablespoon (20 g) raisins or sultanas
500 ml rice or other dairy-free milk

Combine ingredients in a mixing bowl with milk and leave to soak overnight.

FRUIT SALAD

Use any of your favourite berries in this fruit salad for a refreshing start to the day. Choose from blueberries, raspberries, strawberries to some more exotic varieties such as goji, acai or Inca berries. All berries are loaded with vitamin C and powerful antioxidants. Serve on its own or with natural yoghurt. For extra sweetness, drizzle half a teaspoon of raw honey or agave syrup on top.

SERVES 1

½ small banana (35 g), sliced
70 g berries
1 tablespoon sunflower seeds
1 tablespoon pepitas
1 tablespoon almonds
1 tablespoon raisins or sultanas
ground cinnamon, to taste

Mix all ingredients together in a bowl and sprinkle with a pinch of ground cinnamon.

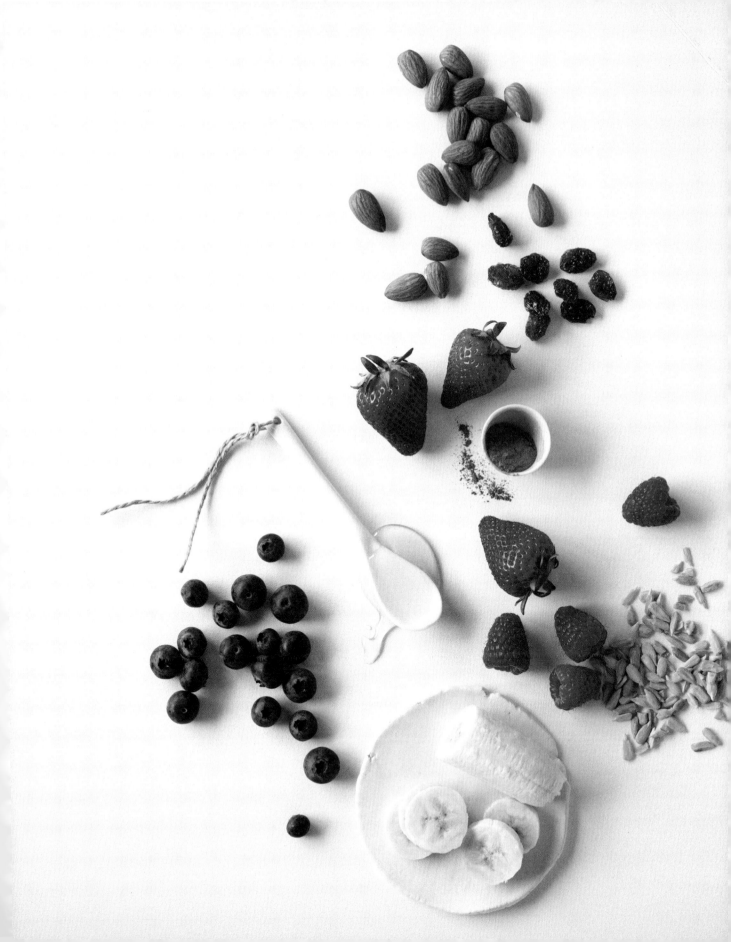

SALMON & ZUCCHINI FRITTATA

This high-protein start to your day is great for detoxing, with its combination of chelating agents, parsley and coriander. To get rid of excess water from the zucchini, grate directly into a large Chux dishcloth and twist until the zucchini is completely dry. If zucchini is not your thing, you can substitute any vegetable you prefer. Serve with a fresh garden salad.

SERVES 4

1 large onion (220 g), roughly chopped
1 clove garlic, minced
⅓ cup (80 ml) extra virgin olive oil, plus extra
　to grease baking dish
10 small zucchini (courgettes) (1 kg), coarsely
　grated and excess water squeezed out
6 large eggs
2 × 85 g tins salmon in spring water
　or brine, drained; flesh, bones and skin mashed
　with a fork
1 tablespoon chopped coriander leaves
1 tablespoon chopped flat-leaf parsley
sea salt and freshly ground black pepper

Preheat oven to 180°C. Grease base and sides of a large baking dish.

Saute onion with olive oil in a large, deep saucepan or small frying pan over medium–high heat until brown (about 5 minutes). Add garlic and zucchini and cook over medium–high heat for 10 minutes, stirring occasionally.

Turn off heat and leave to cool for 20 minutes.

In a mixing bowl, beat eggs lightly with a fork, then add salmon, coriander and parsley. Add zucchini and onion mixture, season with salt and pepper and mix until thoroughly combined.

Pour egg mixture into prepared dish. Bake for 40–45 minutes or until golden brown on top and cooked when tested at centre with a skewer.

Take out of the oven, leave to cool for 10–15 minutes and cut into large slices.

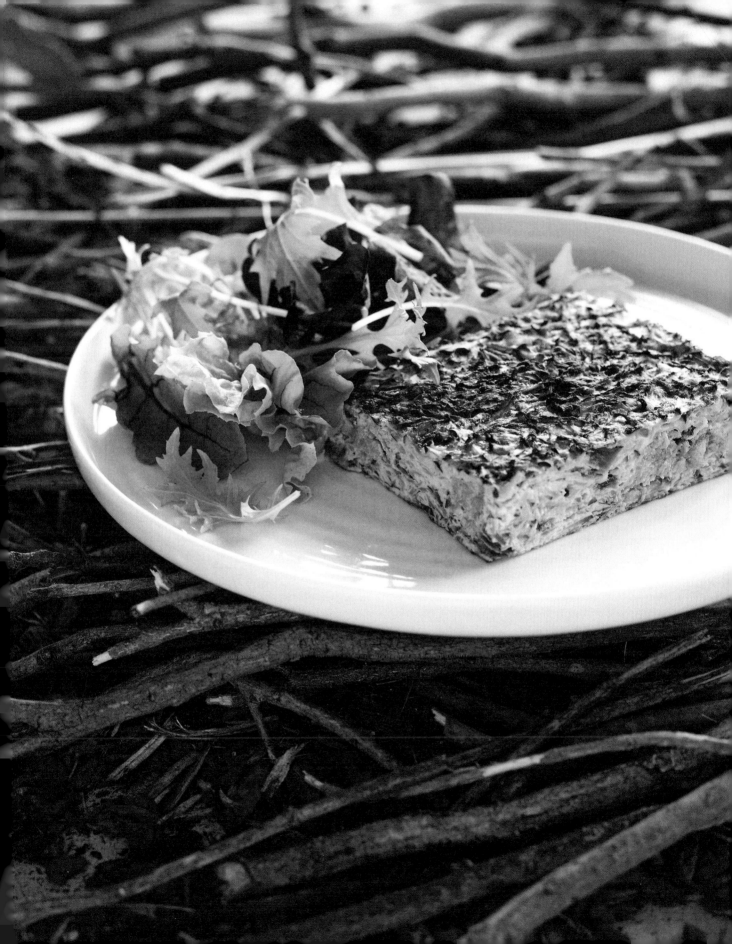

LUNCH

CHICKEN, LEEK & QUINOA RISOTTO

Great for packed lunches as extra portions can be frozen for up to a month. Serve with a rocket salad.

SERVES 2

2 small leeks (200 g)
1 clove garlic, minced
2 tablespoons olive oil
400 g organic chicken breast fillet, cut into
    thin strips
250 ml Vegetable Stock (see p 66) or Radiant Broth
    (see p 95)
2 teaspoons ground coriander
1 tablespoon tomato puree (no sugar)
100 g quinoa
1 tablespoon chopped flat-leaf parsley
juice of ½ lemon
sea salt and freshly ground black pepper

Slice leeks into 1 cm rings, rinse well and pat dry. Saute leeks and garlic in olive oil for 5 minutes then add chicken and cook for a further 10 minutes or till golden.

Pour 250 ml water and stock into a medium-sized saucepan and add cooked chicken mixture, coriander and tomato puree and bring to the boil. Simmer for 5 minutes, and then add quinoa. Simmer for a further 15 minutes or so till water and stock are absorbed. Stir in parsley and lemon juice and season with salt and pepper.

FRESH SPRING ROLLS WITH SESAME SAUCE >

A great one to prepare if you're having friends over as it's fine for your program but they won't know you're detoxing!

SERVES 2

8 × 20 cm rice paper sheets
8 large mint leaves
1 red capsicum (pepper), seeded and thinly sliced
1 carrot, thinly sliced
1 Lebanese cucumber, thinly sliced
½ large ripe avocado, sliced into 8 lengthways
½ cup (50 g) mung bean sprouts
2 teaspoons sesame seeds, toasted

SESAME SAUCE

60 ml wheat-free tamari
1 small clove garlic, minced
½ teaspoon toasted sesame oil
juice of ½ lime
½ teaspoon agave syrup

Submerge the first sheet of rice paper in a large bowl with warm tap water for 5 seconds, then lay on a clean tea towel. Place a mint leaf in centre, then top with a few strips each capsicum, carrot and cucumber and one strip of avocado. Top with some mung bean sprouts.

Fold sides over on to vegetables, and starting closest to you, roll it up. Repeat with rest of sheets, mint and vegetables.

To make sauce, whisk all ingredients together.

Garnish with toasted sesame seeds and serve immediately.

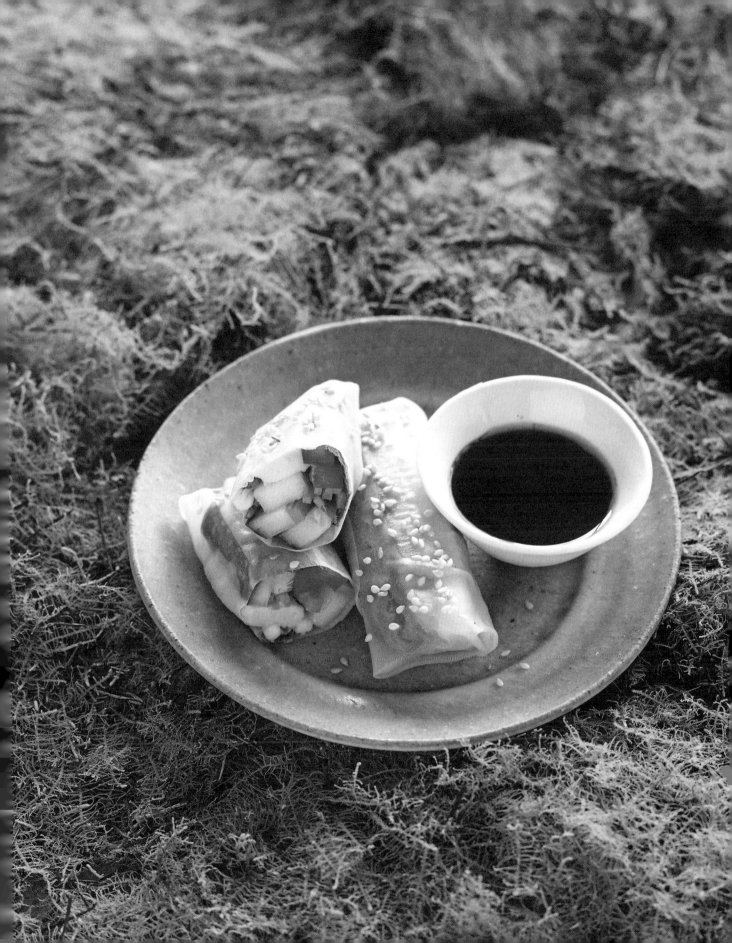

SALAD WITH COCONUT MAYO

This has a nice, creamy texture without any heaviness.

SERVES 2

200 g mixed salad leaves
2 medium tomatoes (300 g), sliced
2 Lebanese cucumbers (260 g), sliced
1 ripe medium avocado (250 g), cut into chunks
1 large carrot (180 g), grated
1 medium beetroot (170 g), peeled and grated
¼ medium red cabbage (300 g), thinly sliced
pepitas and sunflower seeds, to garnish

COCONUT MAYO

1 tablespoon dill, chopped
flesh of 1 young coconut
1 clove garlic
juice of ½ lemon
sea salt
1–2 tablespoons young coconut water

Place all salad ingredients except pepitas and sunflower seeds in a large salad bowl and combine.

To make mayo, place all ingredients except coconut water in a blender, blend on high speed until well combined, then add coconut water as needed to form a creamy consistency.

Pour mayonnaise over salad, fold to combine, then garnish with pepitas and sunflower seeds.

NUT MASH

This is a delicious raw alternative to traditional mashed potatoes - great
served with a piece of grilled fish, chicken, lamb or turkey breast and
a fresh garden salad.

SERVES 4 AS SIDE DISH

35 g macadamia nuts
1 medium–large cauliflower (1.25–1.5 kg),
   trimmed, roughly chopped
1 clove garlic, minced
sea salt
250 ml–300 ml coconut water or almond milk

Soak macadamia nuts in water for
20 minutes, drain and place in a food
processor or blender with cauliflower, garlic
and a teaspoon of sea salt.

Pulse to combine, then with the motor
running, slowly add coconut water or almond
milk until it forms a creamy consistency.

MOROCCAN FISH SKEWERS WITH MILLET SALAD

This wonderfully exotic dish is so scrumptious, you won't believe it is totally fine on a detox. Adding millet to the salad makes for a more filling meal. You can also try the fish skewers with a green salad for a food-combined version. Use any type of low-mercury white fish.

SERVES 4

700 g thick white fish fillets (such as
    barramundi or snapper)
8 bamboo skewers, soaked in cold water
olive oil, for drizzling

MARINADE

1 × 400 g tin crushed tomato
½ teaspoon ground cumin
½ teaspoon turmeric
2 teaspoons paprika
1 teaspoon mild curry powder
2 cloves garlic, finely minced
4 cm piece fresh ginger (20 g), grated
2 tablespoons lime juice

SALAD

200 g hulled millet
1 teaspoon saffron threads
100 g baby spinach
1 red onion, finely chopped
¼ cup flat-leaf parsley leaves, finely chopped
40 g pine nuts, toasted
2 tablespoons olive oil
2 tablespoons lemon juice

Cut fish into large cubes, thread on to skewers and place in a large shallow baking dish. Combine marinade ingredients and pour over fish, coating well. Set skewers aside in the fridge.

To make the salad, add millet to a saucepan with saffron and 625 ml water, bring to the boil over high heat, then turn down the heat to low, cover and simmer for 25 minutes, until all water has been absorbed. Remove from heat, fluff with a fork and allow to cool slightly.

Combine millet with remaining salad ingredients in a large salad bowl and set aside.

Heat oven grill to high, drizzle skewers with a little olive oil, then grill for 2–3 minutes on each side or until just cooked through, then serve with the salad.

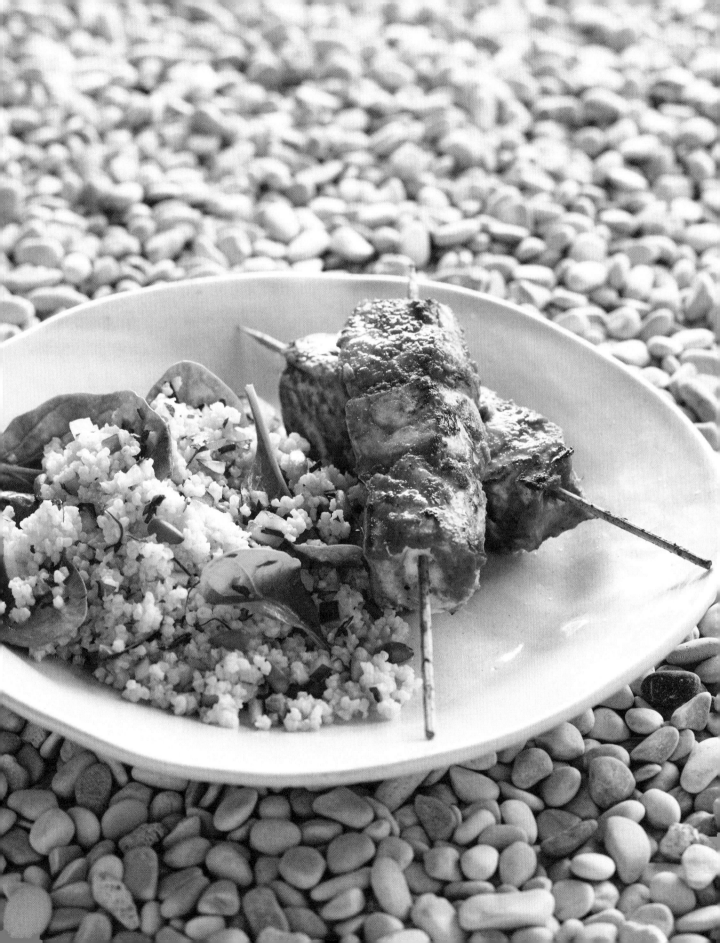

DINNERS

CHICKEN CACCIATORE

A healthy take on this traditional Italian dish. Serve with quinoa, brown rice or some rustic wheat-free bread.

SERVES 4

2 tablespoons olive oil
8 chicken drumsticks
sea salt and freshly ground black pepper
1 red capsicum (pepper)
1 green capsicum (pepper)
1 zucchini (courgette)
1 onion, thinly sliced
2 cloves garlic, minced
½ teaspoon paprika
½ teaspoon chilli flakes
400 ml Vegetable Stock (see p 66)
1 tablespoon raw apple cider vinegar
400 g roma (plum) tomatoes, crushed
2 tablespoons chopped flat-leaf parsley

Heat the olive oil in a large frying pan over medium–high heat. Season chicken with salt and pepper and add to pan. Cook for 10 minutes, turning occasionally, until golden brown and crisp on all sides. Remove from pan and reduce heat to low. Add capsicum, zucchini, onion, garlic, paprika and chilli flakes. Cook for 10 minutes, till vegetables have softened. Add stock, vinegar, tomato and chicken, bring to a simmer, then cover and cook over low heat for about 20–25 minutes, stirring occasionally until chicken is cooked through. Stir in parsley and season with salt and pepper.

ZESTY LAMB CUTLETS

These tasty cutlets are best served with a rocket and cucumber salad, and they're just as good served cold straight from the fridge as a protein snack.

SERVES 4

12 lean lamb cutlets
200 g natural sheep's milk yoghurt
2 cloves garlic, minced
1 teaspoon ground coriander
juice and zest of 1 lemon
½ red onion, finely diced
1 tablespoon chopped flat-leaf parsley
1 tablespoon chopped mint

Combine all ingredients in a large bowl and leave lamb to marinate for 30 minutes. After 20 minutes, preheat grill to medium–high.

Remove lamb cutlets from marinade, discard excess marinade and place the cutlets under grill for 4–5 minutes on each side, turning once, until cooked to your liking.

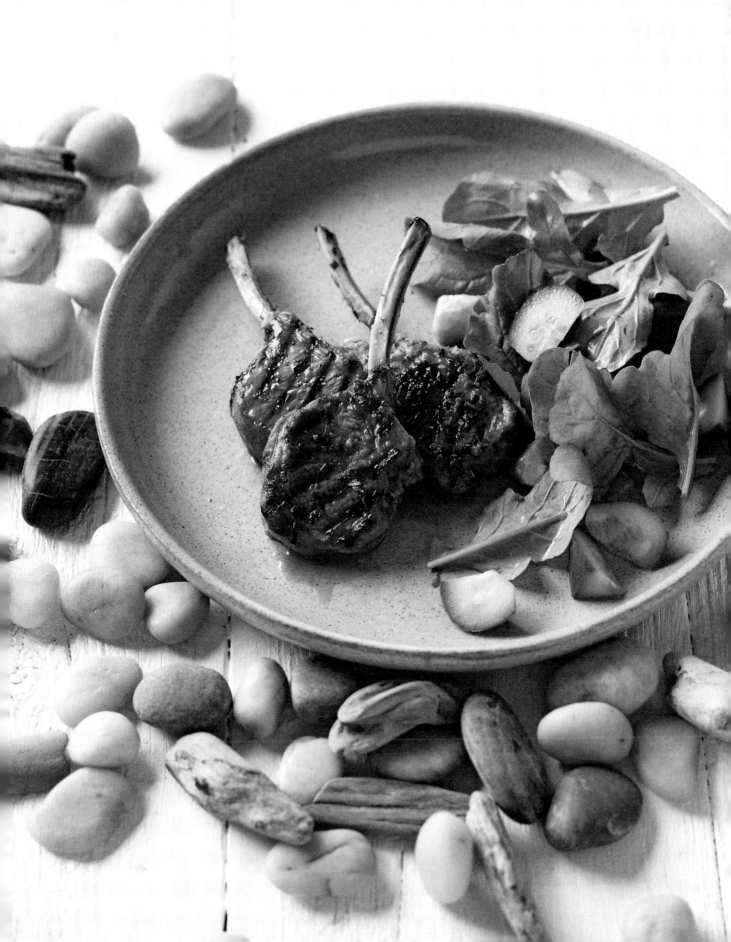

ASIAN-INSPIRED ROAST TURKEY

A fantastic recipe to bake in the oven, or it can be simmered slowly in
a large stockpot or saucepan too. Serve with brown rice or noodles.

SERVES 4

1 tablespoon sesame oil
2 turkey drumsticks
1 green capsicum (pepper) (210 g), seeded and diced
1 red capsicum (pepper) (220 g), diced
1 red onion (175 g), diced
1 white onion (160 g), diced
4 cloves garlic, peeled
1 long fresh green chilli, finely chopped
1 long fresh red chilli with seeds, finely chopped
½ medium Chinese cabbage (600 g), sliced
2 large stalks celery (180 g), diced
1 handful coriander leaves, chopped
1 handful mint leaves, chopped
½ eggplant (215 g), finely chopped
4 cm piece fresh ginger (20 g), grated
1 tablespoon wheat-free tamari
1 tablespoon raw apple cider vinegar
1 × 400 ml tin coconut milk
400 ml water

Preheat oven to 150°C. Combine all
ingredients in a large baking dish (making
sure that vegetables cover turkey to prevent
drying out). Cover with a piece of baking
paper then a doubled piece of foil. Bake for
4 hours or until vegetables and turkey are
very tender and sauce has reduced.

TANDOORI FISH

Serve this with some steamed vegetables tossed with lemon juice and
chopped fresh mint to complete the meal.

SERVES 4

200 g natural sheep's milk yoghurt
2 tablespoons tandoori spice mix
1 clove garlic, minced
¼ cup coriander leaves, chopped
4 × 200 g fillets white fish (such as
    barramundi or snapper)
olive oil, for frying

Place yoghurt, tandoori spice, garlic and
coriander in a mixing bowl, combine well,
then add fish and coat thoroughly with
marinade. Leave to sit for 20 minutes.

Heat olive oil in a frying pan over medium
heat, then add fish and cook for 10 minutes
each side or until just cooked through, and
serve.

SOUPS & BROTHS

LENTIL SOUP WITH GOAT'S CHEESE & GRILLED ZUCCHINI

This hearty soup works well in both summer and winter months, and provides you with lots of energy from the healthy dose of B-vitamins found in lentils.

SERVES 4

1 tablespoon olive oil
1 brown onion, finely chopped
2 stalks celery, trimmed and diced
1 carrot, diced
2 cloves garlic, minced
100 g red lentils
2 × 400 g tins crushed tomato
2 teaspoons ground cumin
1 teaspoon ground coriander
2 tablespoons wheat-free tamari
2 zucchini (courgettes), cut in half lengthways
100 g soft goat's cheese
¼ cup chives, finely chopped

Heat olive oil in a saucepan over medium heat, then add onion and cook until translucent, then add celery, carrot and garlic. Cook for 5 minutes, stirring often, then add lentils, tomato, spices, 500 ml water and tamari. Bring to the boil and simmer for 20 minutes or until vegetables are tender.

Meanwhile, heat grill to high, place zucchini halves, cut-side up, on a baking tray and grill until golden. Combine goat's cheese and chives in a bowl, then spread over grilled zucchini.

Divide soup among bowls and serve each with a zucchini half alongside.

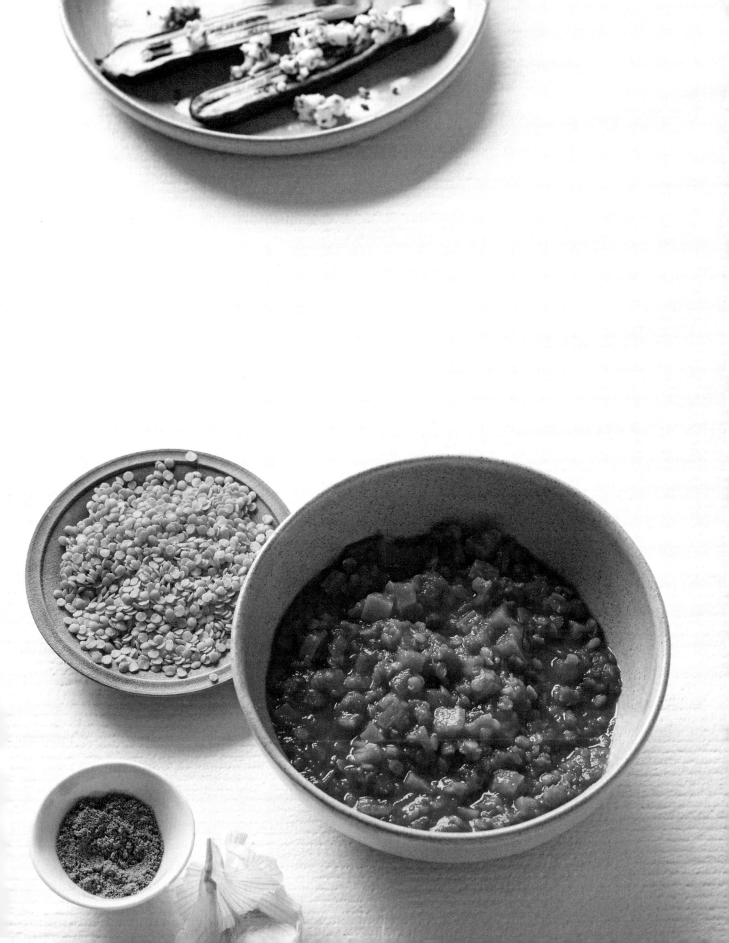

WARMING LAMB STEW

This wonderfully therapeutic stew tastes better the longer you leave it,
and it's incredibly filling too.

SERVES 4

2 cloves garlic, chopped
1 onion, chopped
1 leek, trimmed and cut into 1 cm rings
2 tablespoons olive oil
50 g red lentils
½ teaspoon ground ginger
½ teaspoon ground cumin
½ teaspoon garam masala
½ teaspoon ground black pepper
3 stalks celery, chopped
2 carrots, diced
1 × 400 g tin crushed tomato
500 g diced lamb
50 g brown lentils
1.5 litres Vegetable Stock (see p 66) or Radiant Broth
    (see p 95)
½ cup coriander leaves, chopped
½ teaspoon sea salt

Saute garlic, onion and leek in olive oil in
a large saucepan over medium heat until
translucent. Add lamb and cook for
10–15 minutes. Add garam masala, cumin,
ginger and pepper and cook for a further
5 minutes.

Add celery, carrots, tomato, brown and red
lentils, stock, coriander leaves and sea salt.
Reduce heat to low and simmer for 1 hour.

RADIANT BROTH

The kombu or seaweed is optional – it's included to add extra minerals. Minimum times are given here for simmering, but chicken and fish bones can be simmered for up to 48 hours, and lamb bones for up to 72 hours to extract all the gelatine. The broth will keep for approximately five days in the fridge, or longer if frozen.

MAKES APPROXIMATELY 3.5 LITRES

1–2 chicken carcasses or equivalent fish, or lamb
   bones (about 1 kg)
1–2 tablespoons lemon juice
½ teaspoon dried thyme
½ teaspoon dried oregano
½ teaspoon dried rosemary
2 bay leaves
vegetable scraps (any peelings and ends of organic
   vegetables you happen to have)
1 onion, finely chopped
1 leek, white part only, diced
5 cloves garlic, chopped
1 cup chopped flat-leaf parsley
1 strip kombu seaweed, cut into strips with scissors
80 g chopped cabbage
sea salt and freshly ground black pepper

Put bones, lemon juice and dried mixed herbs in a large stockpot and add enough water to cover completely. Bring to the boil over high heat, then reduce heat to low, cover and simmer for at least 6 hours if you are using chicken or fish bones, and at least 12 hours if you are using lamb bones. To reduce cooking time, cut the bones into small pieces after they have softened a bit (after minimum 2 hours) during cooking. Add more water if necessary to keep bones covered.

Add remaining ingredients except for salt and pepper in the last 2 hours of cooking (or whenever convenient). Skim off any scum that rises to the surface. Add more water as required to keep bones covered (up to 3 litres of additional water may be necessary): you will need at least 3.5 litres of broth remaining.

Remove larger bones from broth with tongs, then strain remainder through a sieve or colander over a large bowl. Press out as much liquid as you can from the scraps, then discard bones and scraps.

Allow broth to cool completely, then skim off any fat on the surface. The cold broth will gel if sufficient gelatine is present, but it won't matter if it doesn't.

To serve, bring to the boil and season with salt and pepper.

CHICKEN SOUP FOR THE SOUL

A healing soup known for its immune-boosting properties. If you enjoy hot spice, a little cayenne pepper is suggested here for extra flavour.

SERVES 4

2 red onions, finely diced
6 cloves garlic, minced
1 teaspoon olive oil
2 litres Vegetable Stock (see p 66) or
    Radiant Broth (see p 95)
4 chicken thigh fillets, skin removed
3 cm piece fresh ginger, peeled
    and finely chopped
1 strip kombu (seaweed), cut into
    1 cm-wide strips
3 stalks celery, finely chopped
200 g cauliflower, chopped
1 carrot, diced
40 g cabbage, finely chopped
40 g kale, roughly chopped
cayenne pepper (optional)
freshly ground black pepper

In a large stockpot, saute onions and garlic with olive oil for 5 minutes. Add stock or broth and 1 litre of water, chicken, ginger and kombu. Cover with a lid and bring to boil over a high heat. Reduce heat to low and add vegetables. Cover with a lid and simmer for 2 hours, stirring occasionally.

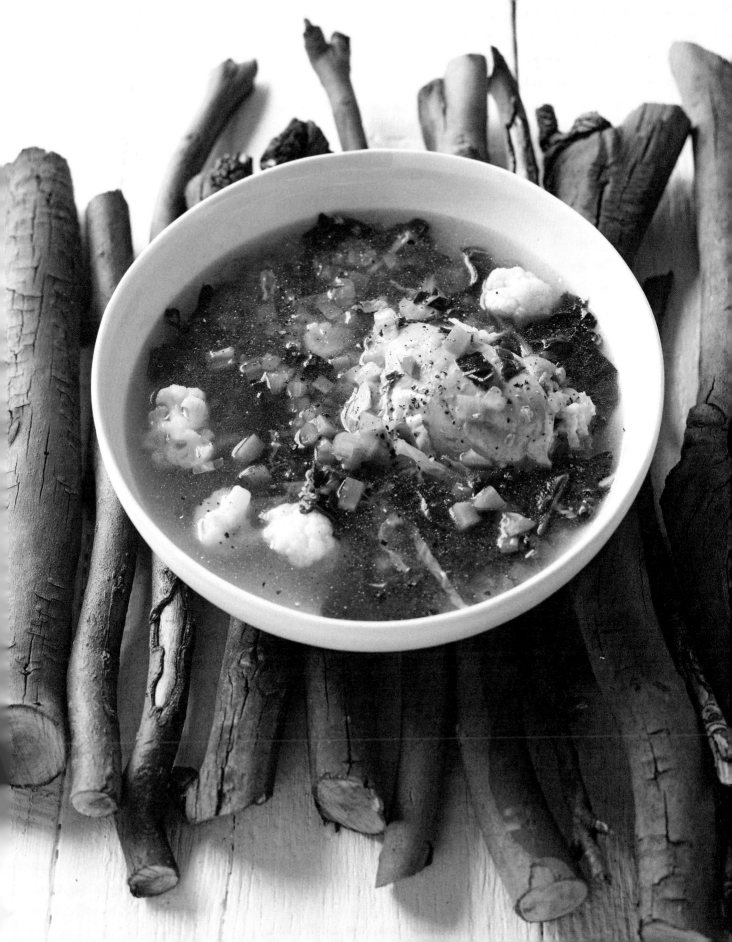

NUTRITIVE PHASE MENU PLANNER – **GENTLE CHART**

	MONDAY	TUESDAY	WEDNESDAY	THURSDAY	FRIDAY	SATURDAY	SUNDAY
On rising	500 ml water Apple cider vinegar–cayenne shot	500 ml water Apple cider vinegar–cayenne shot	500 ml water Apple cider vinegar–cayenne shot	500 ml water Apple cider vinegar–cayenne shot	500 ml water Apple cider vinegar–cayenne shot	500 ml water Apple cider vinegar–cayenne shot	500 ml water Apple cider vinegar–cayenne shot
Breakfast	Easy Bircher Muesli Herbal tea	Cacao-Cashew Smoothie Herbal tea	Fruit Salad Herbal tea	Salmon & Zucchini Frittata Herbal tea	Downward Dog Smoothie Herbal tea	Ancient Grain Porridge Herbal tea	Organic Egg & Zucchini Pancakes Herbal tea
Mid-morning	250 ml Go Green Juice 500 ml water	250 ml Go Green Juice 500 ml water	250 ml Go Green Juice 500 ml water	250 ml Go Green Juice 500 ml water	250 ml Go Green Juice 500 ml water	250 ml Go Green Juice 500 ml water	250 ml Go Green Juice 500 ml water
Lunch	Fresh Spring Rolls with Sesame Sauce	Chicken Soup for the Soul	Tandoori Fish	Moroccan Fish Kebabs with Millet Salad	Chicken, Leek & Quinoa Risotto	Lentil Soup with Goats Cheese & Grilled Zucchini	Radiant Broth
Snacks (only if needed)	500 ml water Handful mixed nuts	500 ml water Crudites with avocado dip	500 ml water Brown rice cakes with tahini	500 ml water Piece of fruit	500 ml water Crudites with hummus dip	500 ml water Rice crackers with avocado	500 ml water 2 tbsps kefir or natural yoghurt
Dinner	Spinach & Seaweed Soup 500 ml water	Asian-inspired Roast Turkey (no grains) 500 ml water	Warming Lamb Stew 500 ml water	Creamy Herb & Cucumber Soup 500 ml water	Radiant Broth 500 ml water	Zesty Lamb Cutlets 500 ml water	Chicken Cacciatore (no grains) 500 ml water
After dinner (optional, only if needed)	1 cup ginger, lemon and honey tea	1 cup peppermint tea with 1 tsp raw honey	2 squares raw cacao chocolate	2 tbsps kefir or natural yoghurt	1 cup peppermint tea with 1 teaspoon raw honey	1 cup ginger, lemon and honey tea	2 squares raw cacao chocolate

NUTRITIVE PHASE MENU PLANNER – **ADVANCED CHART**

	MONDAY	TUESDAY	WEDNESDAY	THURSDAY	FRIDAY	SATURDAY	SUNDAY
On rising	750 ml water Apple cider vinegar–cayenne shot	750 ml water Apple cider vinegar–cayenne shot	750 ml water Apple cider vinegar–cayenne shot	750 ml water Apple cider vinegar–cayenne shot	750 ml water Apple cider vinegar–cayenne shot	750 ml water Apple cider vinegar–cayenne shot	750 ml water Apple cider vinegar–cayenne shot
Breakfast	Algae Drink 300–350 ml Go Green Juice	Algae Drink 300–350 ml Go Green Juice	Algae Drink 300–350 ml Go Green Juice	Algae Drink 300–350 ml Go Green Juice	Algae Drink 300–350 ml Go Green Juice	Algae Drink 300–350 ml Go Green Juice	Algae Drink 300–350 ml Go Green Juice
Mid-morning	750 ml water	750 ml water	750 ml water	750 ml water	750 ml water	750 ml water	750 ml water
Lunch	Algae drink Fish with Fresh Tomato Salsa	Algae drink Stuffed Capsicums	Algae drink Spring Rolls with Sesame Sauce	Algae drink Roast Vegie Salad	Algae drink Tandoori Fish	Algae drink Zesty Lamb Cutlets	Algae drink Salmon Salad with Roast Tomato
Mid-afternoon	750 ml water	750 ml water	750 ml water	750 ml water	750 ml water	750 ml water	750 ml water
Dinner	Algae drink Lentil Soup with Goats Cheese & Grilled Zucchini 750 ml water	Algae drink Simple Avocado Soup 750 ml water	Algae drink Warming Lamb Stew 750 ml water	Algae drink Chicken Soup for the Soul 750 ml water	Algae drink Radiant Broth 750 ml water	Algae drink Spicy Pumpkin Soup 750 ml water	Algae drink Zucchini & Coriander Soup 750 ml water

N.B. Go Green Juice can be drunk either at mid-morning or mid-afternoon

WEEK THREE: MAINTENANCE PHASE

You should be feeling amazing right now and proud of what you have accomplished so far. Your gorgeous, newly alkalised body will be showering you with the gifts of good health – glowing skin, sparkling eyes, lots of energy and a fantastic outlook are all yours to keep.

The Maintenance Phase of the Aussie Body 14-day Diet is about sustaining the good we've done and how to hang on to all the healthful benefits that you've achieved after completing the program. You have transformed yourself on a cellular level, re-ignited your bodily intelligence, revved up your metabolism, and now all you have to do is maintain this sensational feeling.

The easiest principle to follow is '18/21'. If you are having three meals a day, seven days of the week, try to eat alkalising, whole produce for 18 meals in a week. This means you have 1 'free' day per week to eat whatever you feel like. I believe your body can handle this small burden of toxins, because your elimination channels are open and working efficiently, and your vital organs are being given the correct nutrition.

Another way to understand the 18/21 principle is that if you eat healthy, alkalising foods 85 per cent of the time, you can afford to splurge 15 per cent of the time. You will find that when you do, though, your body will show signs of distress much earlier and you will be more attuned to them – simply because you are healthier. For example, when you stop drinking alcohol for a while, if you then have one glass of wine you'll probably feel a bit drunk, and tired and a little lazier the next day because your body is utilising energy to mop up the alcohol. You'll feel the hangover effects because you are meant to experience them – it's your body's way of signalling what is good for you, and what should be reserved for special occasions.

So what to eat 85 per cent of the time? In a nutshell, most of our food and beverage intake should come from unprocessed and alkalising foods, in their whole form. High-quality water, fibre and essential fatty acids should be included in your diet on a daily basis, and processed foods, sugar, wheat, dairy, alcohol and red meat should be reserved for the 15 per cent, as I believe they are acid-forming (please refer to the Acid-Alkaline chart in Guides and Tools, p 196 for a detailed list).

Over the past two weeks whilst doing the program, you may have realised that you actually need far less food than you previously thought. Your portions will probably have become a lot smaller naturally, because of the high volume of liquid in the program – often, when you think you're hungry, you're actually thirsty, so your body will have learned to recognise real hunger more effectively. Moreover, through indulging in the recipes (and making your own up), you'll have realised that food is even better when it is not out of packets and jars and that you don't need all the condiments and sauces you might be accustomed to using when you have access to wonderful herbs and natural flavours. And alkalising, 50 per cent raw foods are easy to prepare, extremely tasty and what's more, they make us feel good after we've eaten them.

Snacks are an option, not a necessity (unless you're running a marathon). Over the past two weeks, you'll have learned to listen to your bodily intuition, which tells you when enough is enough.

Now we'll take this knowledge to the next step in the Maintenance Phase. For example, if you enjoy larger meals in the evenings – say it's your time to sit down together with your family, you enjoy going to restaurants for meals, or you are really busy during the day so look forward to and savour dinner as your main meal of the day, you don't then want to be told to 'breakfast like a king, lunch like a queen, and dine like a pauper', do you? So enjoy your evening meal, but try to have it before 7 p.m. so it doesn't negatively affect your circadian rhythms, and have something lighter to eat for lunch instead.

If you've indulged in the evening, just think about how little time your body has had to use up the energy from the food you have eaten. So if you go on to have a big breakfast the next day and continue this pattern, you might find the kilos will slowly creep on, especially as you age and if you're not exercising sufficiently to use up the energy intake.

The Maintenance Phase is about balance; it's about moving away from restrictions, it's about realising that counting and measuring your food is not sustainable, as it tends to encourage obsessive thoughts about food, rather thinking about the correct balance of food and the quality of your nutrition.

MAINTENANCE TIPS

1 Wherever possible, continue trying to eat organic produce to limit chemical residue entering our bodies and our Earth.

2 Drink at least three litres of pure, high-quality water every day.

3 Brush your skin daily to detox skin, improve circulation and increase lymph flow.

4 Continue to have ACV-Cayenne shot on rising to kick-start digestion and circulation. You can stop this if you wish once you've completed 7 days.

5 If you're an advanced detoxer, keep having an Aloe Drink three times daily 20 minutes before meals during the first week after the 14-day diet (see Liquids for all Phases, p 140 for recipe) to tone the digestive system and serve as an intestinal cleanser.

6 Eat something raw with every meal and try to ensure you are getting 50 per cent raw food – therefore always include a Go Green Juice (preferably at the start of the day), and include fruit, raw vegetables, salads, sprouts, soaked grains,

nuts and seeds and fermented foods with every meal.

7 Add 1 tablespoon of chia seeds or psyllium husks and 1 tablespoon of 'good' oil to your Go Green Juice for your continuing fibre and essential fatty acids needs. You might also want to add 1 tablespoon of micro-algae for a superfood boost.

8 Have one food-combined meal per day – see 'Food Combining Rules' and 'What Is Food Combining?', opposite, for more information. (Advanced: stick to Go Green Juice for breakfast and have one food-combined meal per day.)

9 Make sure you are eating enough protein as this will balance blood sugar levels. See 'Calculate Your Protein Intake' on p 169 and the Protein Estimations table on p 197.

10 Exercise for an hour each day (at least six times per week). Vary the type of activity, intensity and duration. Include cardio as well as conditioning, and at least one yoga session per week. If you need to lose weight, commit to 45 minutes of cardio six times per week.

11 Commit to doing the detox program at least once a year, or twice a year for optimal health. Spring and autumn are the traditional seasons for cleansing the body, but it doesn't matter when, as long as you commit to detoxifying every year for total rejuvenation.

Please note that if you want to lose *more* than six kilograms, it is advisable to do the 14-day gentle detox, followed by one week of maintenance, then move to the 14-day advanced detox, repeating this sequence until you achieve your desired goal weight.

FOOD COMBINING RULES

- Fruit, except melon, should always be eaten with other fruit only, and always 30 minutes before other foods. Don't eat fruit after a food-combined meal.

- All types of melon should only be eaten on their own, not mixed with other fruit.

- Sugary foods should also be eaten alone, before other foods and never straight after a meal. Sugary foods include fruits, syrups, refined sugar, jams and honey.

- Protein and carbohydrates should not be mixed together in the same meal.

- Protein should only be eaten with non-starchy vegetables. Proteins include red meat, poultry, fish, eggs, dairy products, seeds and nuts. Non-starchy vegetables include all except root vegetables, pumpkins and squash.

- Carbohydrates such as breads, rice, pasta, potatoes and legumes should only be eaten with non-starchy vegetables.

WHAT IS FOOD COMBINING?

Food combining is a nutritional approach based on the principle of eating foods that are digested in a similar way together for optimal digestive health. The technique combines specific foods whose components complement one other to enhance nutrient absorption and reduce digestive overload. There are many benefits to be gained from following a proper food-combining diet, including less gas and abdominal bloating after you eat, improved digestion, faster elimination and weight loss or a return to optimal weight.

The theory of food combining is essentially this: proteins require hydrochloric acid and the enzyme pepsin to break them down in the stomach, whereas starches do not start to metabolise until they reach the small intestine, where they require different enzymes for digestion. The environment that starchy foods require is an alkaline one compared to the more acidic one required for protein digestion. Therefore, digestion can be made a much simpler process if foods that require different enzymes, are eaten at different meals. Some foods also are also digested faster and more readily than others. Concentrated proteins may take more than a day to digest, whereas a piece of fruit takes a couple of hours at the most.

When conflicting foods are eaten in combination, the result can be slowed digestion, which leads to ailments such as tiredness or pain after eating; and heartburn or indigestion. Moreover, impaired digestion gives rise to fermentation of foods in the gut and putrefaction. This in turn feeds pathogens such as candida. Naturopaths believe these harmful bacteria then makes our bodies more acidic, which promote further growth. As a result of the tilt in our body's ecosystem, beneficial bacteria are compromised, and this is when disease starts to set in.

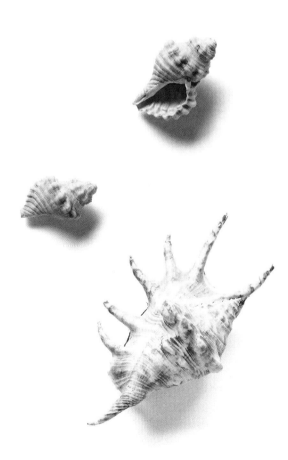

POST-DETOX FAQ

Can I go back to having my daily coffee? You absolutely can, but really try to limit it to just one as it's an acid-forming food that can play havoc with the body. Make sure you're not drinking it on an empty stomach. This mucks up blood sugar levels, enticing us to eat sweets in the afternoon, and puts unnecessary stress on our adrenals.

Will I put the weight I've lost back on again? You won't as long as you follow the 18/21 rule (see p 100) and commit to doing a detox two or three times a year. If you're still concerned, try a weekly one-day cleanse – one day per week eating a very light diet, or having only juices and soups in order to give your digestion a rest and allow the body to detoxify itself. This weekly ritual will promote the elimination of build-up and is extremely beneficial for continued weight loss.

Also eat three meals a day with limited snacking (only if you're actually hungry, not bored!). The body needs time to process each meal, and the digestive system needs a rest between meals. If you are constantly snacking, your system does not have time to fully process one meal before it has to start work on the next. Naturopaths believe that constant grazing causes the accumulation of toxins.

And stick to the rules of eating 50 per cent raw, and having at least one food-combined meal per day. Drink lots of water.

Do I need to continue with all of my supplements? It depends on what your needs are and where the imbalances in your body are. It is a great idea to consult with your naturopath, but as a rule of thumb, if you are healthy and eating a mainly organic diet, taking moderate exercise and keeping your stress levels low, having a Go Green juice with extra fibre in the form of chia seeds or psyllium husk and some essential fatty acids is all you need for optimal health.

Any tips for eating out? Enjoy eating out and stick to the 18/21 rule (you can halve your free day into two half-days if you really must). Remember that food generally tastes better in restaurants because it is laden with butter, fat, condiments, salt and sugar. The healthier you become, the more you will notice this, along with the quality of produce.

Stick to the food-combining rules and fill up on lots of vegies and salad. If it's night time, lose the bread, pasta, rice, tortilla and naan bread. Try to begin with a salad, and finish with a digestive tea such as ginger, peppermint or fennel.

Any tips for alcohol consumption? Unfortunately, champagne, white wine and beer are the main culprits for digestive problems including bloating. If you have a tendency to digestive problems, avoid these completely and stick to spirits (these have most of the yeast burnt off in the process). No sugary mixers, just fresh lime and soda – or neat on ice!

How can I speed up my metabolism? Cayenne pepper, chilli, ginger and green tea raise your body temperature, which increases your metabolism. And there is no substitute for exercise.

Can I ever party again? Of course you can! The fantastic thing about cleaning our bodies on a regular basis is that when we do want to party or go through periods of indulgence, our bodies respond better. First, the bad news – you'll feel the effects of over-consumption a little more and this is simply because you are now used to feeling 100 per cent, so feeling 75 per cent feels like you're being cheated.

Secondly, the good news – remember that we are here to enjoy our lives, and that means from time to time, we enjoy indulging and should never, ever feel guilty about it. By cleansing the body on a regular basis, we naturally balance out any harm we've done and what's more, we are also naturally not as excessive, and therefore reach a happy medium. The partying eventually stops when you have an alkalised body, because you will be itching to feel 100 per cent again.

| CASE STUDY |

VICTORIA ALEXANDER, *writer and photographer*

'When was the last time you felt light?' came the question from my wonderful son-in-law. It had been a while.

My reason for visiting Saimaa was primarily to lose the weight that had slowly crept on. It was just after an extended period of muscular pain in my legs, caused by heart medication, and up-and-down thyroid function which had eaten into my exercise resolve. I had become used to working so late into the night that I would hear the birds' welcome in the morning, I had no set mealtimes, and I was skipping the odd meal.

Keen to detox after seeing a friend look so great I embarked on a six-week program. In the beginning I was given so many tablets I felt I might begin to rattle, and was told to be in bed by 11 p.m. each night.

The program included eating every three to four hours, I found myself thinking 'Oh God! I've got to eat again.' I lost a kilo a week and loved doing so. The continuing three litres of water every day makes my brain feel clear.

The effect was immediate. I had no cravings and now more than three months later my resolve is set. I have a way of eating that makes me want to keep at it because it feels so damn good. I've lowered my cholesterol and it is great to feel in balance.

Saimaa's encouraging manner helped me to take up yoga, something I had been meaning to do. Detoxing is now a way of life. One I do not intend to part with as the reward is in the doing and the resolve to stay on track makes me feel perfectly smug. You know when you are on the right track when others ask for the detox doctor's number.

MAINTENANCE PHASE RECIPES

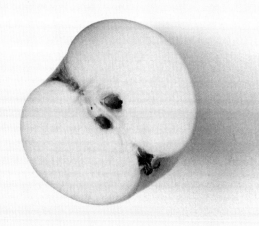

BREAKFAST

LUNCH

DINNER

SWEET TREATS

BREAKFAST

SCRAMBLED TOFU & VEGIES

A spicy take on a popular vegan breakfast dish. Serve on its own or with toast.

SERVES 2

¼ red onion, finely chopped
1 clove garlic, minced
1 green capsicum (pepper), diced
1 red capsicum (pepper), diced
65 g cherry tomatoes, halved
1 tablespoon extra virgin olive oil, plus extra
    for drizzling
250 g organic firm tofu, crumbled
½ fresh bird's eye chilli, finely chopped
½ teaspoon ground cumin
½ teaspoon ground coriander
1 teaspoon wheat-free tamari
small handful of coriander leaves
sea salt and freshly ground black pepper

Saute onion, garlic, capsicum and tomato in the tablespoon of olive oil in a frying pan for about 5 minutes over a medium heat. Add tofu, chilli, spices, tamari and coriander and stir to combine well with onion mixture. Cook for 10 minutes, stirring well. Season with salt and pepper and serve with a drizzle of extra virgin olive oil.

GOAT'S CHEESE, SPINACH & MUSHROOM OMELETTE >

This popular omelette is being served more frequently in healthy cafes and restaurants. It is high in protein and very filling. Serve on its own or with a rocket salad.

SERVES 1

2 eggs
20 g goat's cheese
1 clove garlic, minced
¼ red onion, finely chopped
½ bunch spinach, finely chopped
¼ tomato, finely chopped
4 button mushrooms, finely chopped
1 tablespoon fresh or dried oregano
2 tablespoons olive oil
sea salt and freshly ground black pepper

Crack eggs into a mixing bowl and whisk till light and fluffy. Add all other ingredients to the bowl and mix thoroughly.

Heat olive oil in a frying plan on medium heat. Pour omelette mixture into pan and cook for 3–5 minutes, until just cooked through. Season with salt and pepper and serve.

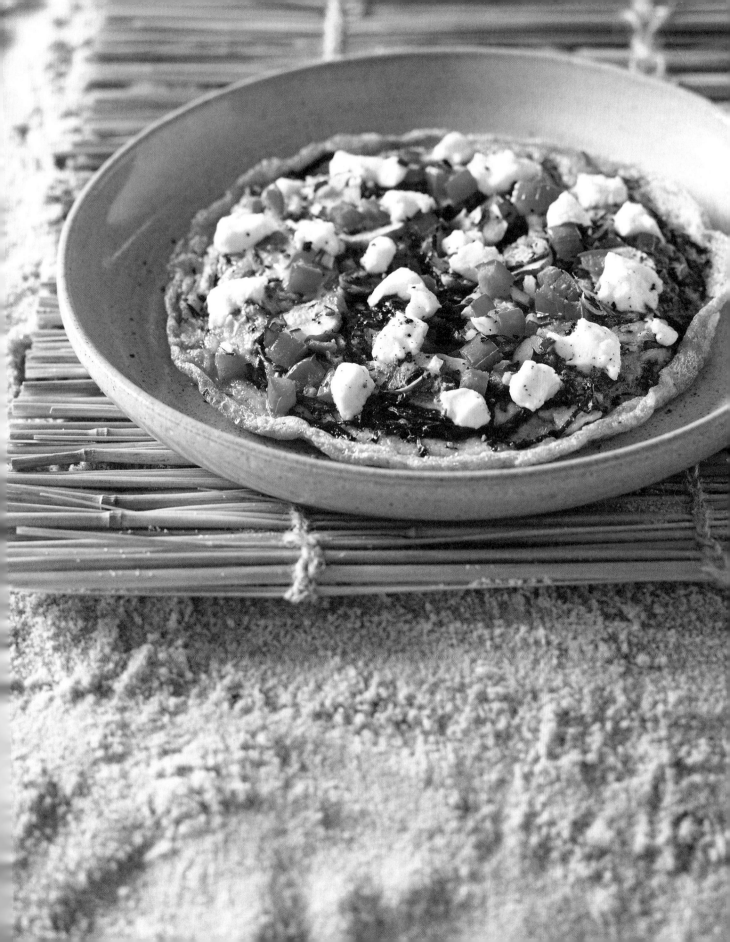

BERRYLICIOUS PORRIDGE

Berries are nutritional powerhouses, chock-full of antioxidants,
and are simply delicious. Vary the taste of this porridge by using different
berries – from blueberries, raspberries, blackberries and strawberries
through to goji (or wolfberry), Inca (or golden berry), acai, sumac and
many other amazing varieties. Serve with a sprinkle of cinnamon
on top or with one or two tablespoons of natural yoghurt.

SERVES 1

90 g rolled oats
1 tablespoon oat bran
250 ml any dairy-free milk such as nut,
    seed, oat, rice or quinoa milk
150 g berries (for example blueberries,
    raspberries, and/or strawberries)
½ medium banana (100 g)
1 tablespoon chia seeds

In a small saucepan over medium heat,
combine oats and oat bran with milk and
250 ml water, stirring well. Bring to boil, then
reduce heat to low and simmer for a further
5 minutes until oats are thick and creamy.
Remove pan from heat and stand for 1 minute.
Spoon porridge into a bowl and serve with
berries, banana and chia seeds.

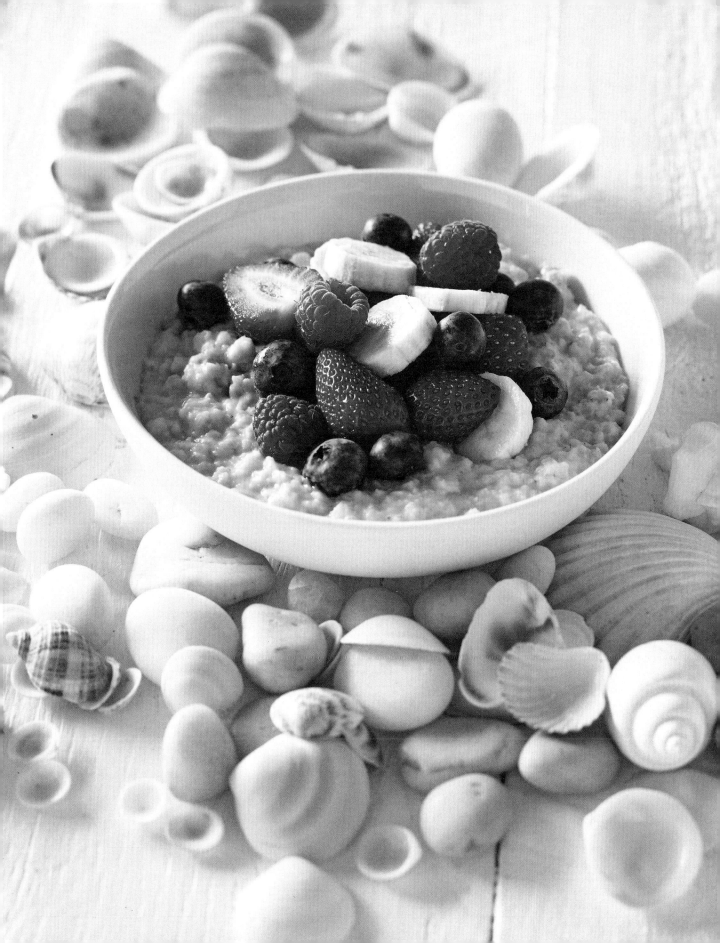

LUNCH

HERB-INFUSED LAMB & BEAN SALAD

This recipe uses lemon-infused flaxseed oil, which you can buy from gourmet delicatessens or make by paring the rind from an organic lemon, covering with oil and leaving to infuse for a few days.

SERVES 4

60 ml olive oil
1 teaspoon dried oregano
1 teaspoon dried rosemary
small pinch cayenne pepper
juice of ½ lemon
2 cloves garlic, minced
4 × 300 g lamb backstrap, trimmed
sea salt and freshly ground black pepper
200 g green beans, trimmed
1 small green cucumber, thinly sliced
2 spring onions, thinly sliced
¼ cup finely chopped mint
¼ cup finely chopped flat-leaf parsley
200 g goat's cheese, crumbled
2 tablespoons lemon-infused flaxseed oil
4 lemon wedges

Place olive oil, herbs, lemon juice, and garlic in a bowl and stir to combine. Add lamb and mix until well coated, then season with salt and pepper, cover and chill for 1 hour.

Blanch the green beans in boiling water for 5 minutes, then place them with all remaining ingredients except lemon wedges in a salad bowl and toss to combine.

Pan-fry lamb over high heat for 3–4 minutes each side for medium–rare, or continue until cooked to your liking. Slice thinly and serve warm on the salad with the lemon.

ROAST VEGIE SALAD >

A favourite with guests. Complements any type of meat dish too.

SERVES 4

4 baby beetroots
500 g butternut pumpkin, peeled and cut into
   3 cm chunks
4 cups baby spinach
2 Lebanese cucumbers, cut into thin ribbons
   with a vegetable peeler
1 spring onion, thinly sliced
30 g walnut pieces, cut into quarters
1 tablespoon flaxseed oil
1 tablespoon raw apple cider vinegar
100 g goat's cheese

Preheat oven to 220°C.

Trim and wash beetroot, leaving skin on. Wrap beetroot in foil, place on a baking tray and bake for 40 minutes. Remove tray from oven, add pumpkin and return to oven for a further 20 minutes. When cool enough to handle, rub skin off beetroot.

Place spinach, cucumber and spring onion in a large salad bowl and add beetroot and pumpkin, tossing to combine well. Add walnuts, oil and vinegar and combine. Crumble goat's cheese over top and serve.

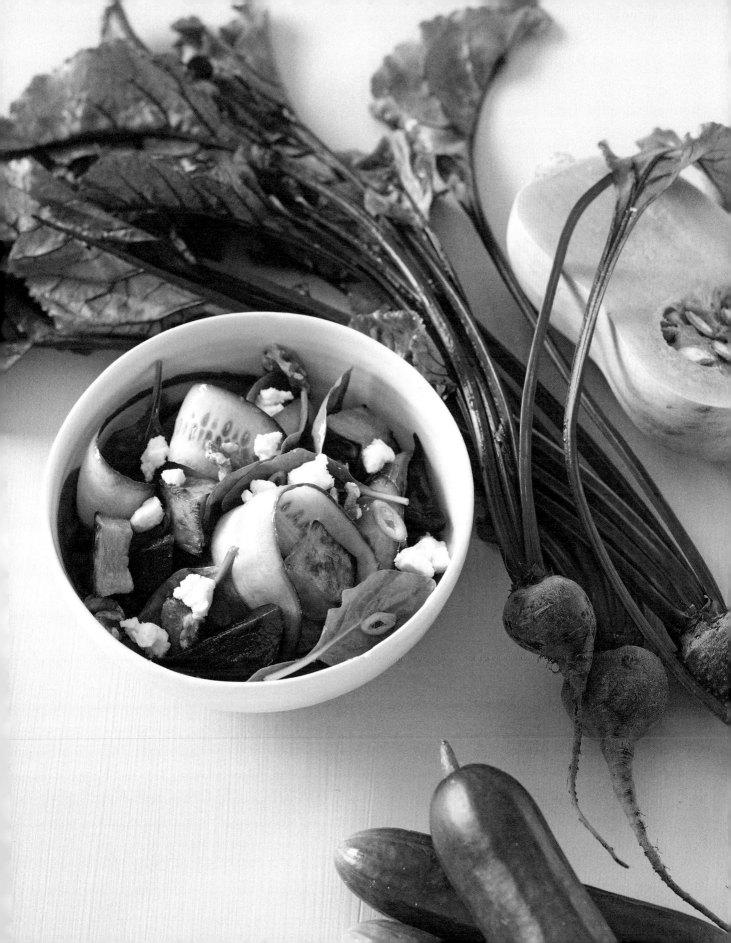

SALMON & CORIANDER PESTO PILAF

This Persian-inspired dish is full of powerhouse nutrients, and uses the coriander pesto dip from Extra Goodies for all Phases on p 130. Adjust the amount of coriander pesto to your taste.

SERVES 4

2 teaspoons olive oil
1 onion, finely chopped
2 cloves garlic, minced
2 teaspoons finely grated lemon zest
300 g medium-grain brown rice
1 tablespoon raw apple cider vinegar
700 ml vegetable stock
250 g broccoli, cut into small florets
70–80 g coriander pesto, to taste
100 g baby rocket leaves
1 × 150 g smoked salmon fillet, skin removed and coarsely flaked

Heat olive oil in a saucepan over medium heat, then add onion and cook, stirring, for 5 minutes until translucent. Add garlic and lemon zest and cook for 1 minute until fragrant.

Add rice and stir for 2 minutes until grains start to turn translucent. Add vinegar and stock and bring to the boil.

Stir once, then cover, turn the heat down to low and cook for 35 minutes. Remove from heat, place broccoli florets on top of rice and replace lid. Leave to steam for 5–10 minutes until broccoli is tender and bright green.

Fluff rice, stir through coriander pesto and rocket. Serve topped with salmon.

WASABI SALMON SALAD >

The wasabi dressing gives this a Japanese twist. Leave out the fruit if you don't want to combine sweet and savoury.

SERVES 2

1 beetroot
2 × 200 g salmon fillets
olive oil, for drizzling
sea salt and freshly ground black pepper
150 g mixed salad leaves, torn
1 apple, cored and thinly sliced
1 ripe avocado, cut into 2 cm dice
2 tablespoons pepitas
2 tablespoons sunflower seeds
1 tablespoon flaxseed, ground
2 tablespoons goji berries

WASABI DRESSING

2 tablespoons raw apple cider vinegar
1 teaspoon wasabi
juice of 1 lime
¼ cup (60 ml) extra virgin olive oil

Preheat oven to 180°C. Cook beetroot in a saucepan in just enough boiling water to cover for 1–1½ hours, until you can pierce it easily with a skewer. Cool slightly, rub off skin and cut into 2 cm dice.

To make dressing, place vinegar, wasabi and lime juice in a blender. Blend on medium for 30 seconds. Switch to lowest setting and slowly pour in oil with the motor running.

Drizzle salmon with a little olive oil and season. Cover with foil, then bake on a baking tray for 15 minutes.

Put salad leaves in a large bowl and toss. Sprinkle with remaining ingredients. Lightly 'lift' with your fingers to distribute greens. Use a fork to flake salmon into bite-sized pieces. Arrange on top and drizzle with dressing.

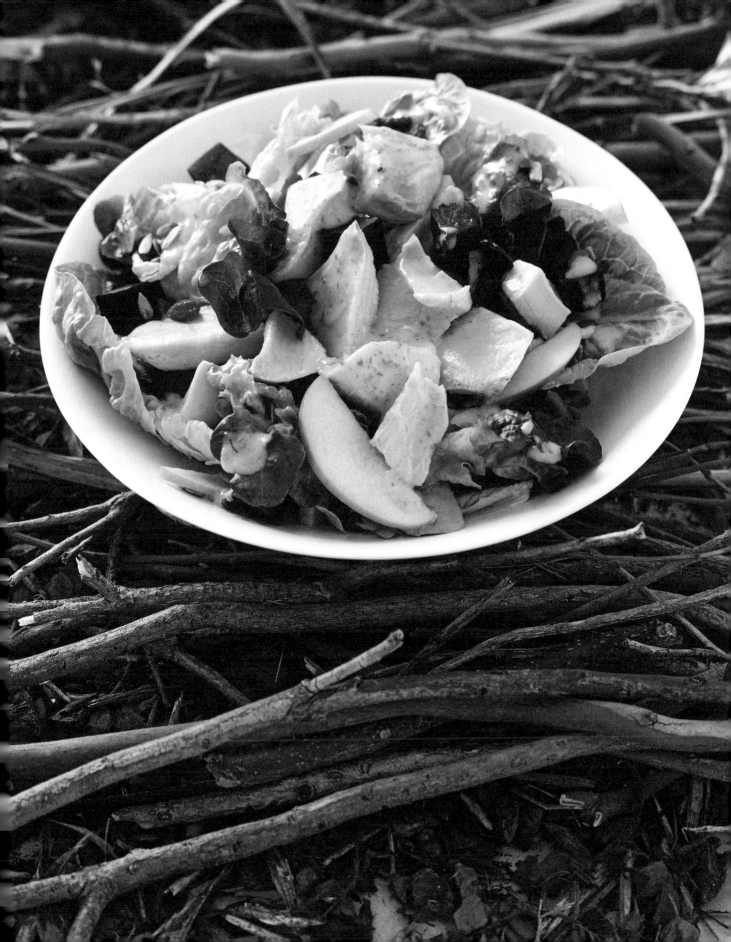

DINNER

CHICKEN TORTILLA

If you're having this dish in the detoxification phase, choose a yeast-free, gluten-free tortilla or flat bread.

SERVES 2

350 g skinless chicken tenderloins
1 tablespoon olive oil
1 teaspoon chilli powder
1 teaspoon ground cumin
sea salt and freshly ground black pepper
6 corn tortillas
4 fresh green chillies
1 medium red onion (150 g), sliced
150 g mixed salad leaves

GUACAMOLE

1 ripe medium avocado (150 g), stone removed
juice of 1 lime
1 clove garlic, minced
2 tablespoons finely chopped coriander
small pinch paprika

Preheat oven to 120°C.

Preheat chargrill pan over medium–high heat. Coat chicken with olive oil, rub spices in and season. Place tortillas in oven to warm.

Cook chicken, chilli and onion in grill pan for 4–5 minutes on each side until firm and slightly charred. Turn chillis and onion often and remove from heat when chicken is ready.

To make guacamole, scoop avocado into a bowl, add the rest of the ingredients and mash until combined.

Serve chicken in tortillas with guacamole, grilled vegetables and salad leaves.

CHIMICHURRI STEAK

Chimichurri always accompanies grilled steak in Argentina. It is also perfect as a marinade for beef or chicken.

SERVES 2

350 g sirloin or rump steak
sea salt and freshly ground black pepper
olive oil, for frying
½ bunch cavalo nero (black kale), thinly sliced

CHIMICHURRI SAUCE

½ cup chopped flat-leaf parsley
4 cloves garlic, minced
1 teaspoon fresh or dried oregano leaves
½ teaspoon chilli flakes
60 ml raw apple cider vinegar
1 teaspoon lemon juice
2 tablespoons water
60 ml olive oil
½ teaspoon sea salt
freshly ground black pepper

To make the chimichurri, place all ingredients in a food processor or blender and pulse to combine.

Heat a frying pan over high heat. Season steak with salt and pepper, add a little olive oil to the pan and cook steak for 3–4 minutes on each side for medium–rare (or to your liking). Keep the heat turned on and place steak on serving plate.

Add cavalo nero to pan, sprinkle over a tablespoon of water and cook, stirring often, for 2–3 minutes until slightly wilted.

Slice steak thinly, drizzle with chimichurri sauce and serve cavalo nero alongside.

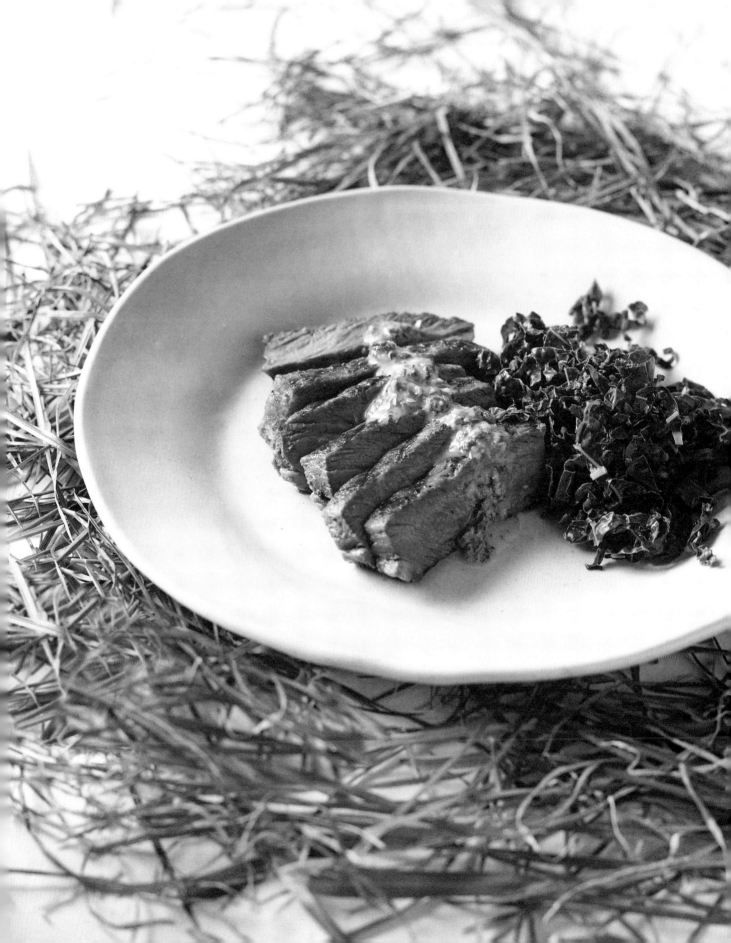

HEARTY LAMB SHANKS

A great one for the slow-cooker, so you can prepare it in the morning
and arrive home after work to find it ready. Serve on its own.

SERVES 2

2 × 250 g lamb shanks
2 stalks celery, diced
1 brown onion (150 g), diced
2 carrots, diced
1 parsnip, diced
1 turnip, diced
1 swede, diced
1 potato, diced
1 bulb garlic, cloves separated
1 × 375 g tin crushed tomato
2 tablespoons wheat-free tamari
1 tablespoon raw apple cider vinegar
50 g pearl barley
1 handful flat-leaf parsley, roughly chopped

Place lamb shanks in the base of a slow
cooker. Add all vegetables.

Place garlic cloves in a bowl and cover with
boiling water. Allow to soak for 2 minutes,
then drain, peel the skins off and add the
garlic cloves to slow cooker.

Add tomato, tamari, vinegar and barley.
Cover with water. Put lid on and set dial to
auto. Cook on low heat and check after
6 hours. The meat should fall off the bone;
this can take up to 8 hours.

SUCCULENT OSSO BUCO

A healthy take on this traditional Italian dish.

SERVES 4

2 pieces beef shin (700 g)
1 brown onion, diced
1 carrot, diced
1 potato, diced
300 g kent pumpkin, peeled and diced
1 green capsicum (pepper), diced
1 long fresh red chilli, finely chopped
4 tomatoes, diced
4 spinach leaves, shredded
300 g green cabbage, thinly sliced
4 large sage leaves
1 handful chopped flat-leaf parsley
2 × 15 cm sprigs rosemary, leaves stripped
2 bay leaves
6 cloves garlic, peeled
1 tablespoon wheat-free tamari
1 tablespoon agave syrup
1 tablespoon tomato paste
100 g medium-grain brown rice

Preheat oven to 150°C (or 130°C with fan assistance). Combine all ingredients in a 6-litre capacity, heavy-based baking dish with lid (making sure that vegetables cover beef to prevent drying out) and add enough water to cover. Cover with a round piece of baking paper. Bake for 6 hours or until vegetables, rice and beef are very tender and sauce has reduced. Stand covered for 15 minutes before serving.

SWEET TREATS

RAW CACAO MOUSSE

This unusual recipe uses an avocado to create a creamy, silky texture, and is delicious served with fresh berries.

SERVES 4

2 ripe bananas, peeled
1 avocado, peeled, seeded and cut into chunks
1 tablespoon raw cacao powder
1 tablespoon raw cacao nibs
1 teaspoon agave syrup
2 teaspoons iced water

Place all ingredients in a small food processor with 2 teaspoons iced water and blend until it reaches a smooth, creamy consistency. Spoon into serving glasses and chill for at least 2 hours before serving.

MACA MAGIC BALLS >

Raw maca, from Peru, is touted as a superfood for its wonderful composition of protein, vitamins and minerals, and is thought to enhance strength and endurance. These make a great afternoon snack or after-dinner sweet, and can be stored in an airtight container in the fridge for up to two weeks. Kids love them too.

MAKES AROUND 20 BALLS

60 ml agave syrup
5 fresh medjool dates (115 g), pitted
125 g ground almonds
2 tablespoons raw cacao powder
1 teaspoon raw maca powder
1 tablespoon coconut butter
20 g desiccated coconut, for rolling

Place all ingredients except desiccated coconut in a food processor and blend until well combined and mixture sticks together. Scoop out mixture a tablespoon at a time and use your hands to roll into balls, then finish them off by rolling in coconut.

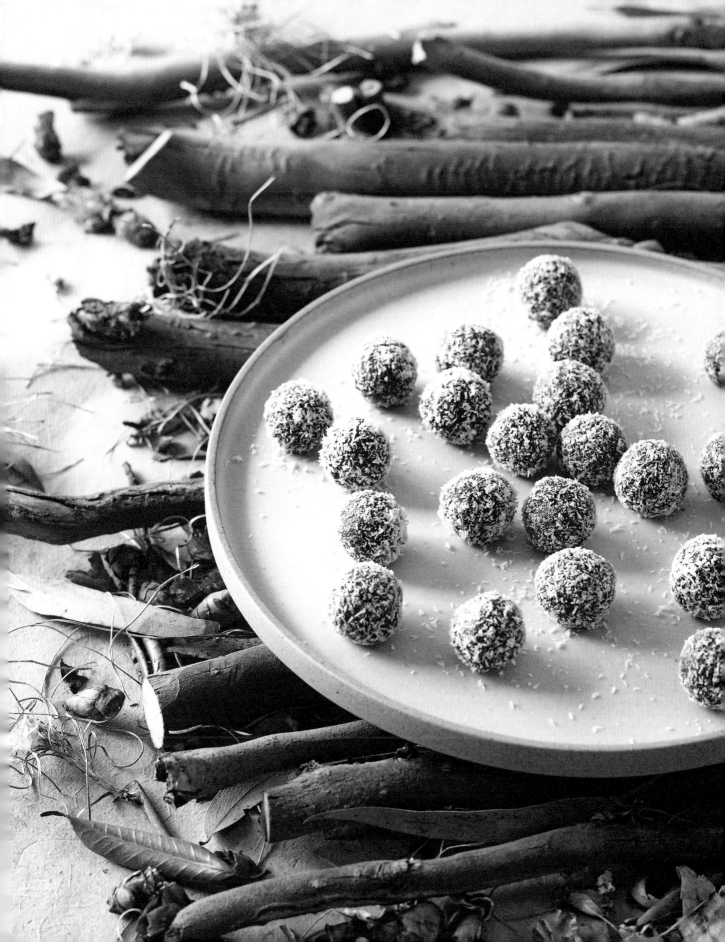

BANANA MUFFINS

These are wonderful served warm from the oven, but any you don't eat straight away can be kept in an airtight container for up to three days. They also freeze well for up to a month.

MAKES 10 MUFFINS

150 g rice flour
75 g arrowroot
1 teaspoon baking powder
1 teaspoon cream of tartar
2 eggs, lightly whisked
75–100 ml rice milk
1 tablespoon coconut butter, melted
2 ripe bananas (350g), mashed

Preheat oven to 190°C. Grease 10 holes of a 12-hole (⅓-cup capacity) muffin tray.

In a medium-sized mixing bowl, combine rice flour, arrowroot, baking powder and cream of tartar.

Beat eggs, rice milk, coconut butter and mashed bananas in another medium-sized bowl. Fold in the flour mix, then stir using a fork until just combined; do not overmix – mixture should still look lumpy.

Spoon mixture into greased muffin pan, filling each hole three-quarters full (approximately 2 heaped tablespoons in each).

Bake for 18–20 minutes or until a skewer inserted in the centre comes out clean. Rest in tray for 3 minutes, then remove to a wire rack to cool.

NO-BAKE COOKIES >

A favourite for the sweet-toothed, chock-full of nutrients and fibre. You can use chopped nuts to coat the cookies if you prefer.

MAKES 8-10 COOKIES

200 g raw almonds
10 fresh medjool dates, pitted
2 tablespoons (30 g) chia seeds
20 g desiccated coconut, plus extra for coating
40 g sunflower seeds
40 g pepitas (pumpkin seeds)
25 g raw cacao powder
1 tablespoon agave syrup
2 tablespoons unhulled tahini
60 ml unsweetened apple juice

Place almonds in food processor and blend until roughly ground. Add dates, chia seeds, coconut, sunflower seeds, pepitas and cacao powder. Blend again, then add syrup and tahini, blending until well combined. With the motor still running, slowly pour in apple juice and blend until the mixture forms a thick consistency.

Scoop out 1 tablespoon of mixture at a time, roll into balls and flatten into rounds. Coat with coconut or chopped nuts as desired, and store any you don't use straight away in an airtight container in the fridge for up to a week.

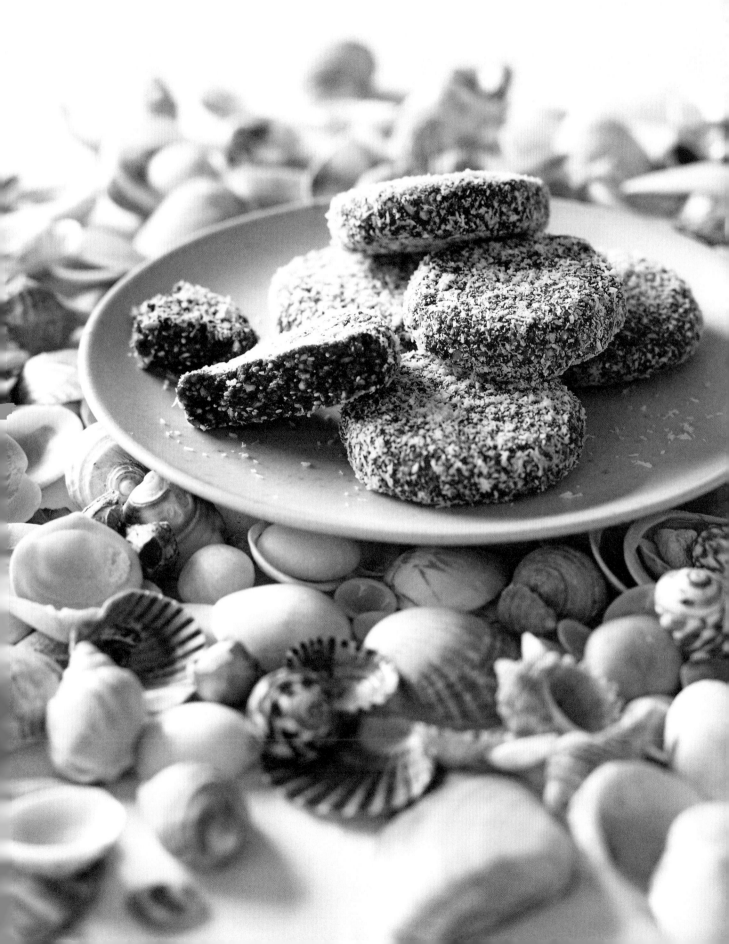

TAMARILLO & APPLE RAW CRUMBLE

A deliciously tangy take on the traditional crumble. Serve on its own or with natural yoghurt.

SERVES 4

80 g sunflower seeds
80 g seeded medjool dates, chopped
50 g walnuts
½ teaspoon ground ginger
sea salt
3 large apples (600 g), grated
40 g dried unsweetened cranberries
1 teaspoon ground cinnamon
2 cloves, ground
2 tamarillos, cut into wedges

Preheat oven to 100°C.

In food processor or blender, process first sunflower seeds, then add dates, followed by walnuts, ginger and a pinch of salt. Blend until mixture is the consistency of fine crumbs and well combined. Transfer to a bowl and set aside.

Process half the grated apple with cranberries, cinnamon, ground cloves and a pinch of salt until it forms a smooth consistency.

In a large bowl, combine tamarillo, remaining apple and blended apple mixture together. Pour into a shallow glass or ceramic oven dish and sprinkle seed mixture evenly over the top. Place dish in the oven and warm for 45 minutes before serving.

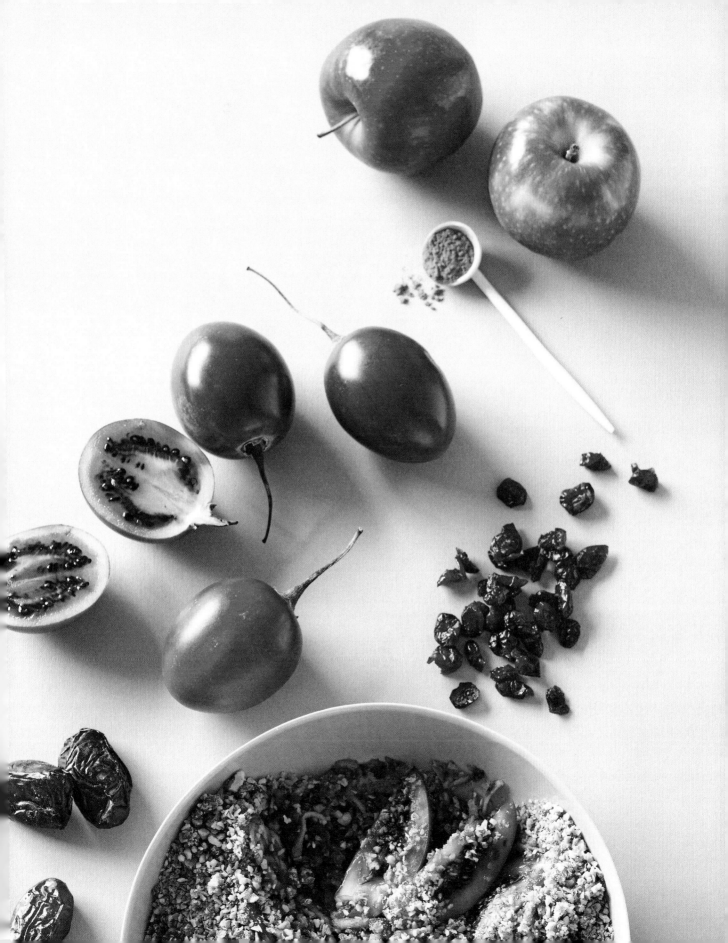

RAW BERRY ICE-CREAM

If you have an ice-cream machine, making this ice-cream will be very
simple, but don't worry if not – you'll just need to take it out of the
freezer and re-blend with a stick blender every couple of hours.
Raspberries, blueberries and strawberries all work well in this recipe, and
it's lovely served with fresh berries.

SERVES 6–8 (MAKES 1 LITRE)

150 g raw cashews, soaked overnight
10 fresh medjool dates, pitted
250 ml almond milk (or other dairy-free milk)
125 g raspberries, blueberries or strawberries
1 small banana, peeled
60 g coconut butter, melted
80 ml agave syrup
juice of ½ lemon
1 teaspoon pure vanilla extract
sea salt

Drain and rinse cashews, place in a blender
or food processor with remaining ingredients
and blend until well combined and a smooth,
creamy consistency.

Transfer mixture to a 2-litre plastic container
and place in freezer. Take it out every 2 hours
and re-blend using a stick blender until
you're happy with the texture – it usually
takes about 8 hours. Alternatively, churn and
freeze in an ice-cream machine according to
manufacturer's instructions.

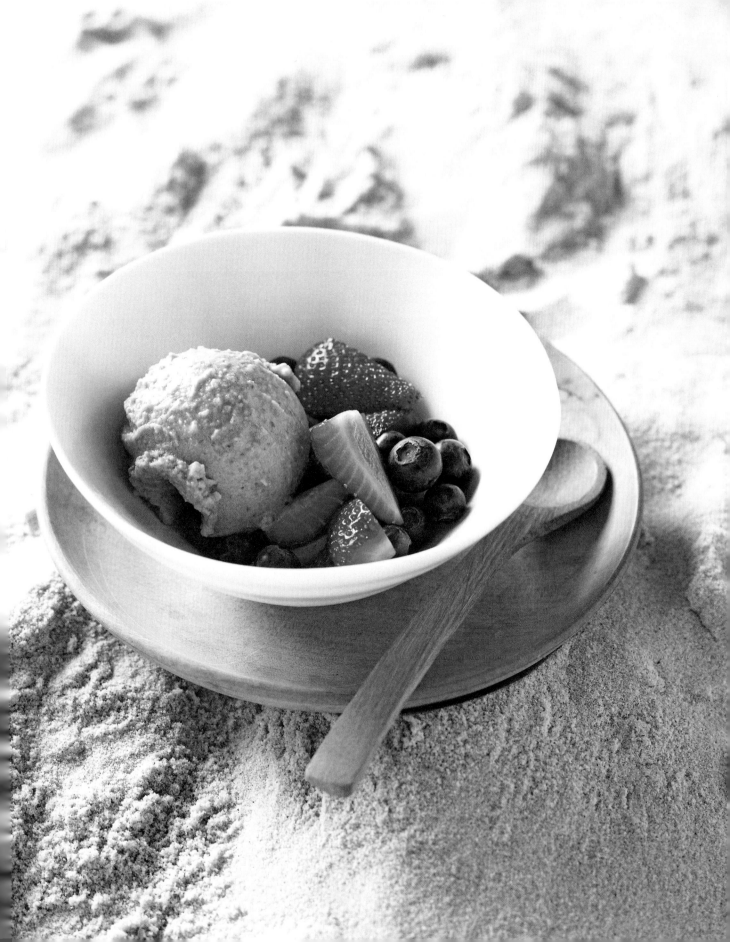

MAINTENANCE PHASE MENU PLANNER – **GENTLE CHART**

	MONDAY	TUESDAY	WEDNESDAY	THURSDAY	FRIDAY	SATURDAY	SUNDAY
On rising	750 ml water Apple cider vinegar–cayenne shot	750 ml water Apple cider vinegar–cayenne shot	750 ml water Apple cider vinegar–cayenne shot	750 ml water Apple cider vinegar–cayenne shot	750 ml water Apple cider vinegar–cayenne shot	750 ml water Apple cider vinegar–cayenne shot	750 ml water Apple cider vinegar–cayenne shot
Breakfast	Aloe drink Green drink	Aloe drink Green drink	Aloe drink Green drink	Aloe drink Green drink	Aloe drink Green drink	Aloe drink Green drink	Aloe drink Green drink
Breakfast	Berrylicious Porridge 750 ml water	Goat's Cheese, Spinach & Mushroom Omelette 750 ml water	Scrambled Tofu & Vegies 750 ml water	Banana-Berry Smoothie 750 ml water	Salmon & Zucchini Frittata 750 ml water	Cacao-cashew Smoothie 750 ml water	Organic Egg & Zucchini Pancakes 750 ml water
Lunch	Wasabi Salmon Salad	Roast Vegie Salad	Moroccan Fish Kebabs with Millet Salad	Salmon & Coriander Pesto Pilaf	Asian-inspired Roast Turkey	Energy Soup	Herb-infused Lamb & Bean Salad
Mid-afternoon	750 ml water Handful mixed nuts	750 ml water Crudites with avocado dip	750 ml water Brown rice cakes with tahini	750 ml water Piece of fruit	750 ml water Crudites with hummus dip	750 ml water Rice cracker with avocado	750 ml water 2 tbsps kefir or natural yoghurt
Dinner	Chicken Tortilla 750 ml water	Chimichurri Steak 750 ml water	Spinach & Seaweed Soup 750 ml water	Hearty Lamb Shanks 750 ml water	Spicy Pumpkin Soup 750 ml water	Succulent Osso Buco 750 ml water	Tandoori Fish 750 ml water
After dinner (optional, only if needed)	Raw Cacao Mousse	1 cup peppermint tea with 1 teaspoon raw honey	Maca Magic Balls	2 tbsps kefir or natural yoghurt	No-bake Cookies	Ginger, lemon and honey tea	Raw Berry Ice Cream

MAINTENANCE PHASE MENU PLANNER – **ADVANCED CHART**

	MONDAY	TUESDAY	WEDNESDAY	THURSDAY	FRIDAY	SATURDAY	SUNDAY
On rising	750 ml water Apple cider vinegar–cayenne shot	750 ml water Apple cider vinegar–cayenne shot	750 ml water Apple cider vinegar–cayenne shot	750 ml water Apple cider vinegar–cayenne shot	750 ml water Apple cider vinegar–cayenne shot	750 ml water Apple cider vinegar–cayenne shot	750 ml water Apple cider vinegar–cayenne shot
Breakfast	Aloe drink 300–350 ml Go Green Juice	Aloe drink 300–350 ml Go Green Juice	Aloe drink 300–350 ml Go Green Juice	Aloe drink 300–350 ml Go Green Juice	Aloe drink 300–350 ml Go Green Juice	Aloe drink 300–350 ml Go Green Juice	Aloe drink 300–350 ml Go Green Juice
Mid-morning	750 ml water	750 ml water	750 ml water	750 ml water	750 ml water	750 ml water	750 ml water
Lunch	Aloe drink Scrambled Tofu & Vegies	Aloe drink Roast Vegie Salad	Aloe drink Moroccan Fish Skewers with Millet Salad	Aloe drink Salmon & Coriander Pesto Pilaf	Aloe drink Radiant Broth	Aloe drink Goat's Cheese, Spinach & Mushroom Omelette	Aloe drink Buckwheat Pancakes (with wilted spinach and cherry tomatoes)
Mid-afternoon	750 ml water	750 ml water	750 ml water	750 ml water	750 ml water	750 ml water	750 ml water
Dinner	Aloe drink Wasabi Salmon Salad 750 ml water	Aloe drink Warming Lamb Stew 750 ml water	Aloe drink Chicken Soup for the Soul 750 ml water	Aloe drink Herb-infused Lamb & Bean Salad 750 ml water	Aloe drink Chicken Cacciatore 750 ml water	Aloe drink Hearty Lamb Shanks 750 ml water	Aloe drink Lentil Soup with Goat's Cheese & Grilled Zucchini 750 ml water

N.B. Go Green Juice can be drunk either at mid-morning or mid-afternoon

AUSSIE BODY
14-DAY DIET

EXTRA GOODIES
FOR ALL PHASES

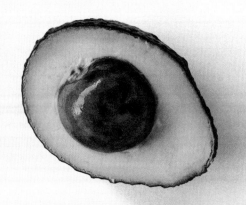

EXTRA GOODIES

EXTRA GOODIES

KEFIR

Kefir is a fermented milk drink made by adding fresh milk to kefir grains. It contains essential amino acids, magnesium and calcium. Studies show it can improve the digestion of lactose in lactose-intolerant people. Loaded with beneficial bacteria, it's also a natural immunity-booster, and has both prebiotic and probiotic qualities. Only use glass or plastic equipment when making kefir; it is important to avoid using metal implements as they interact with the enzymes and render them inactive.

MAKES 350 ML

1–2 tablespoons fresh kefir grains or ½ tablespoon freeze-dried kefir grains
350 ml fresh goat or sheep milk

Place kefir grains in a sterilised 500 ml glass jar, pour in milk and cover with a clean cloth.

Leave to stand at room temperature for approximately 24 hours. Kefir is ready when the liquid congeals and solids begin to separate.

When ready, stir the mixture, then strain, using a glass or plastic strainer, into a glass or plastic bowl. Use a plastic funnel to transfer the kefir into a glass bottle and store in the refrigerator; it is now ready to drink.

Place the kefir grains in a separate glass jar with a little milk and store at room temperature, topping it up regularly to keep them alive.

Experiment with the amount of kefir you add and the fermentation times to achieve your favoured taste and consistency. The longer the kefir is left to ferment the thicker and more sour in taste it will become.

SAUERKRAUT

This age-old dish boasts many healing properties due to its high concentration of probiotics. The longer you leave it, the more sour it will become. It will ferment faster at higher temperatures. If any surface mould appears, scrape it away and discard along with any discoloured sauerkraut.

MAKES 4–5 KG

4–5 kg organic cabbage at room temperature – green, purple or a mixture
¼ cup sea salt, rock salt or Himalayan crystal salt, dried and ground
1 tablespoon caraway seeds

Set aside a couple of whole leaves, then cut the rest into quarters and remove core. Shred cabbage finely using a food processor or knife.

Place cabbage in a large bowl, sprinkle over the salt and caraway seeds, then massage and squeeze cabbage with your hands until it starts to soften and liquid appears.

Pack cabbage into a sterilised 2-litre glass jar or ceramic crock, then use your fists or a wooden utensil to pack the cabbage down tightly until the liquid has risen to the top and all the cabbage is submerged.

Cover top of cabbage with whole cabbage leaves and weight with pastry weights (or the cabbage core, or some tins of food); this seals it so it can ferment without air. Drape a cloth over the top to keep flies away.

Leave at room temperature for approximately 2 weeks, tasting at regular intervals.

Store covered in the refrigerator; it will keep for at least 3 months.

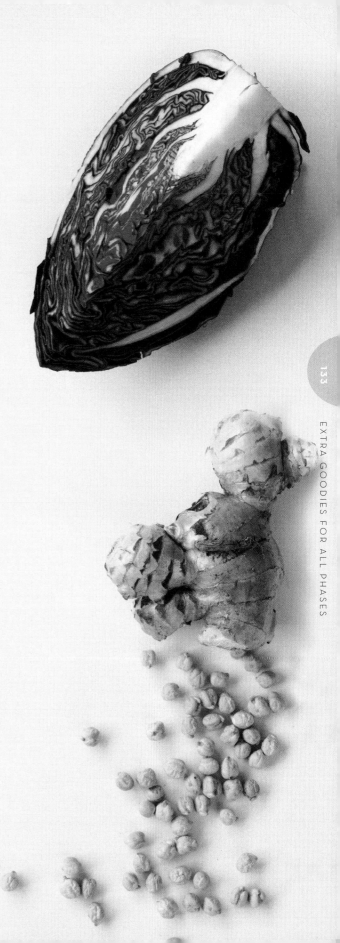

RAW FERMENTED VEGETABLES

You can be creative with your choice of vegetables and flavour combinations – this recipe is just a guide.

MAKES 4 KG

3 green cabbages, cored and shredded, a few whole
    leaves reserved
6 large carrots, shredded
7 cm fresh ginger, roughly chopped
6 cloves garlic, roughly chopped

Combine all ingredients except for reserved cabbage leaves in a large bowl. Put 2 cups of mixture in a blender along with 250 ml filtered water, then blend well, add back into the bowl and stir to combine.

Pack vegetables into a sterilised 2-litre glass jar or ceramic crock, using your fists or a wooden utensil to pack the vegetables down tightly until the liquid has risen to the top and all of the vegetables are submerged.

Cover with whole cabbage leaves and press down with pastry weights (or the cabbage core); this seals the vegetables so they can ferment without air. Drape a cloth over top of jar to keep flies away.

Leave at room temperature for at least three days, tasting regularly; the longer it ferments, the stronger the flavour will be.

Store, covered, in the refrigerator; it will keep for at least 3 months.

HEAVENLY HUMMUS

A heavenly take on this traditional Middle Eastern dip – and fine on a detox!

MAKES 750 ML

2 × 400 g tin chickpeas, drained and rinsed
3 cloves garlic, minced
80 ml tahini
½ teaspoon sea salt
½ teaspoon freshly ground black pepper
½ teaspoon ground cumin
½ teaspoon paprika
juice of 2 lemons
80 ml flaxseed oil

Place all ingredients in a blender or food processor with 60 ml filtered water and blend until creamy. Add more water if you want a thinner consistency.

Serve immediately or store in a container in the refrigerator for up to a week.

CREAMY AVOCADO DIP

The flavour of this dip intensifies if it is covered and placed in the refrigerator for a few hours before serving. To help prevent it from turning brown on top, simply place an avocado stone in with the dip while chilling, then remove it before serving.

MAKES 500 ML

2 large avocados, halved and stones removed
juice of 1 lime
1 clove garlic, minced
1 tablespoon finely chopped red onion
1 small tomato, seeded and diced
½ teaspoon sea salt
½ teaspoon freshly ground black pepper
small handful coriander leaves, finely chopped

Scoop out avocado flesh, place in a bowl and mash with a fork. Add remaining ingredients and mix well to combine.

Can be served immediately, or refrigerated for a few hours to develop the flavours.

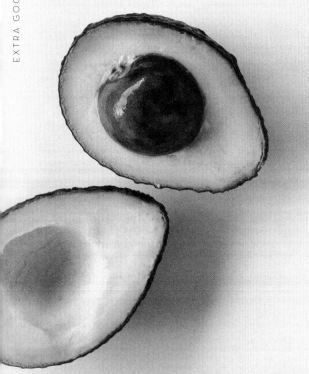
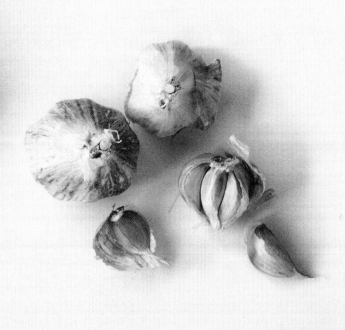

ROAST GARLIC AIOLI

This immunity-boosting dip serves as a delicious accompaniment to many savoury dishes.

MAKES 1 CUP

10 cloves garlic
1 organic egg yolk
1 teaspoon wholegrain mustard
1 cup (250 ml) olive oil
1 tablespoon lemon juice

Preheat oven to 160°C.

Place unpeeled garlic cloves on a baking tray and roast for 10–15 minutes until tender. Once cooled slightly, squeeze garlic out of skins and set aside to cool completely.

Put egg yolk and mustard into a blender, and, with the motor running, add olive oil in a very slow stream, then add lemon juice. Keep blending for a few seconds, then add the cooled, roasted garlic and blend until just combined.

Serve immediately or store in a glass container in the refrigerator for up to a week.

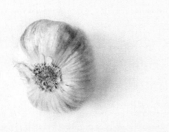

KITCHARI

Kitchari is based on Ayurvedic cleansing principles and is said to draw toxins from deep in the tissues. It is made from mung dahl, a favourite in Ayurvedic medicine as it is easy to digest. I have included it as an excellent source of vegetarian protein. It is very nourishing, yet light. You can adjust the amount of water according to how liquid you'd like it to be, and vary the spices according to taste.

SERVES 2

½ cup (100 g) yellow mung dahl (lentils) or sprouted whole mung beans
½ cup (100 g) white basmati rice or quinoa (brown rice can be used but must be soaked first)
1 teaspoon ghee
½ teaspoon mustard seeds
½ teaspoon cumin seeds
½ teaspoon ground cumin
½ teaspoon ground coriander
½ teaspoon turmeric
1 pinch asafoetida
4 cm piece fresh ginger (20 g), chopped
250 g chopped vegetables (optional – try carrot, cabbage, beetroot, greens or sweet potato)
sea salt to taste
fresh coriander, to taste (optional)
lime halves (optional)

Soak lentils (and if you're using brown rice, soak that too) for 2 hours before cooking. Wash lentils and rice together 2 or 3 times.

Heat ghee and mustard seeds in a large saucepan over medium heat until seeds begin to pop. Add remaining spices and ginger and cook for 2 minutes, stirring constantly. Add rice and lentils and stir to coat with spice/ghee mix. Add 250 ml water. Add vegetables, if using. Bring to a boil and cook for 15 minutes or until rice and lentils are soft. You may need to add more water. Season with salt and garnish with coriander and/or lime.

TZATZIKI

It's best to start this the day before to really drain the yoghurt and cucumbers.

MAKES 625 ML

560 g natural sheep's milk yoghurt
2 telegraph cucumbers
½ teaspoon sea salt
60 ml olive oil
2 cloves garlic, minced
½ teaspoon freshly ground black pepper
1 teaspoon dill, finely chopped

Place yoghurt in a sieve lined with muslin over a bowl and leave to drain in the fridge for at least 2 hours or preferably overnight.

Halve cucumbers lengthways, scoop out seeds and discard, grate flesh and place in a colander. Sprinkle with salt and leave in fridge for at least 15 minutes, but preferably overnight, then squeeze out excess liquid.

Place yoghurt, cucumber and remaining ingredients in a bowl and mix well to combine.

CORIANDER PESTO

Coriander enhances the detoxifying qualities of this traditional pesto dip.

MAKES 375 ML

2 cups fresh coriander leaves, rinsed and dried
½ cup (75 g) macadamias
¼ cup (40 g) pine nuts
¾ cup (180 ml) olive oil
1 clove garlic, minced
juice of 1 lemon
½ teaspoon sea salt
1 teaspoon kelp powder

Place all ingredients in a blender or food processor and blend to a creamy consistency. Serve immediately or store in a glass jar in the refrigerator, with a thin layer of olive oil on top to prevent oxidation, for up to a week.

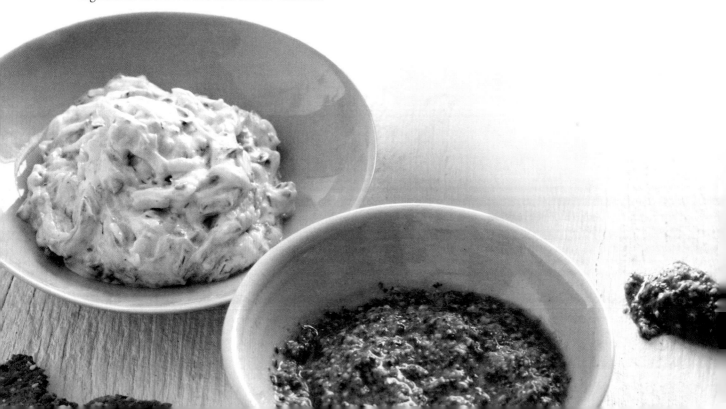

RED CAPSICUM DIP

A colourful and flavoursome dip served with crackers or vegie sticks.

MAKES 500 ML

2 large red capsicums (peppers), cored, deseeded
    and roughly chopped
50 g walnuts
75 g cashews
2 cloves garlic, minced
juice of 1 lemon
½ teaspoon sea salt
½ teaspoon freshly ground black pepper
½ fresh red birds-eye chilli, seeded and
    finely chopped
½ teaspoon ground cumin

Place all ingredients in a blender or food processor with 125 ml water and blend until creamy. Serve immediately or store in a glass container in the refrigerator for up to a week.

SEED & NUT CRACKERS

These gluten-free crackers are delicious and go with all the dips in this chapter.

MAKES ABOUT 20 CRACKERS

35 g wholegrain spelt flour, plus extra
35 g buckwheat flour
30 g ground almonds
½ teaspoon sea salt
2 teaspoons kelp powder
40 g sunflower seeds
2 tablespoons sesame seeds
2 tablespoons linseeds
2 tablespoons olive oil

Preheat oven to 180°C and line 2 baking trays with baking paper.

Mix all dry ingredients together until well combined. Add oil and 125 ml water and mix; add water as necessary until the dough just comes together. If it gets too sticky add extra flour by the teaspoonful until desired consistency is reached.

Roll out dough until 5 mm thick on a floured sheet of baking paper with a well-floured rolling pin.

Place on baking trays and bake for 15–20 minutes or until crackers are just starting to colour. Place on a cooling rack and break into pieces when cool.

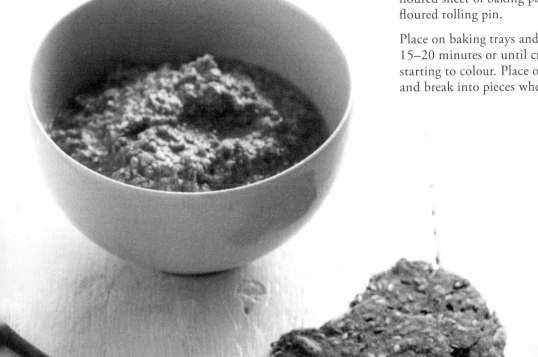

LIQUIDS
FOR ALL PHASES

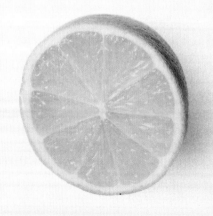

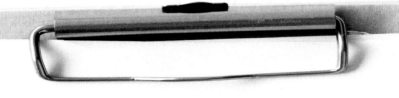

REMEDIES

JUICES

SMOOTHIES

NUT & SEED MILKS

TEA

REMEDIES

APPLE CIDER VINEGAR & CAYENNE SHOT

Raw apple cider vinegar is alkalising, helps with weight loss and may help delay the onset of type 2 diabetes. Opt for apple cider vinegar made from doubly-fermented whole apples; it should not be distilled, filtered or pasteurised as doing so can destroy important nutrients. Raw and organic is always best. Cayenne pepper is warming, stimulates your circulation and can aid in weight loss. It's best to take this remedy on rising, 15 minutes before having a Go Green Juice or breakfast. Adjust the amount of warm water you use according to taste – some people can tolerate a stronger solution, while others need it to be more diluted.

SERVES 1

1 teaspoon raw apple cider vinegar
1 pinch cayenne pepper
50–100 ml warm water, to taste

Mix together and drink.

ALGAE DRINK

The Algae Drink is to be drunk three times daily during the Nutritive Phase. For the algae powder, choose from either a ready-made mix (such as Udo's Beyond Greens or Vital Greens), or a single algae such as spirulina or dunaliella salina.

SERVES 1

1 teaspoon algae powder
1 teaspoon chia seeds or psyllium husks
100 ml water, lime-infused water or
    fresh coconut water

Mix well (make sure the algae powder is completely mixed in) and drink.

ALOE DRINK

The Aloe Drink should be drunk three times daily during the Maintenance Phase. Aloe vera has traditionally been used as a powerful intestinal membrane cleanser and aids in toning the digestive system with its soothing and anti-inflammatory qualities.

SERVES 1

1 tablespoon aloe vera juice
1 teaspoon chia seeds or psyllium husks
100 ml water, lime-infused water
    or fresh coconut water

Mix well and drink.

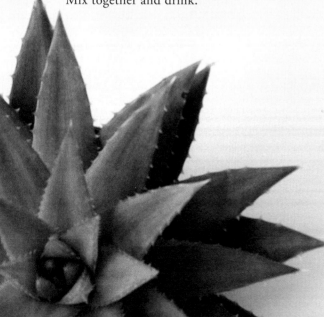

DETOX DRINK

Detox Drink should be drunk three times a day during the Detoxification Phase. The psyllium husks give you fibre, which is important to help bind toxins and eliminate them effectively. Fibre also cleans the digestive tract and helps to build immunity. Psyllium husks are a super form of soluble fibre that attracts water and swells into a gel, helping bulk up faeces and relieve constipation. Research shows psyllium husks may lower 'bad' blood cholesterol levels. Sprinkle them on cereal or stir into a glass of water; drink immediately before it thickens.

Bentonite clay, available from health food shops, has been used for centuries for its purifying qualities, helping to draw out toxins. It is one of the most effective natural intestinal detoxifying agents. It can also be used on the skin as a face mask or applied all over the body. Liquid Bentonite clay can be purchased from most health food shops and health spas or order online at websites such as iherbs.com or healingclays.com.au.

Coconut water has had a resurgence in popularity in recent times but again, people have been drinking it for centuries. Fresh coconut water (from a young coconut, not bottled) provides the body with electrolytes, minerals and essential fatty acids. It also makes the Detox Drink taste more pleasant, and is very hydrating. It is optional, however, and you can use filtered water or lime-infused water (put a couple of slices of lime in a jug of water and leave to infuse for at least 30 minutes).

SERVES 1

1 teaspoon chia seeds or psyllium husks
1 tablespoon of liquid or edible bentonite clay
100 ml water, lime-infused water, or fresh
    coconut water

Mix well (make sure the clay is thoroughly dissolved) and drink.

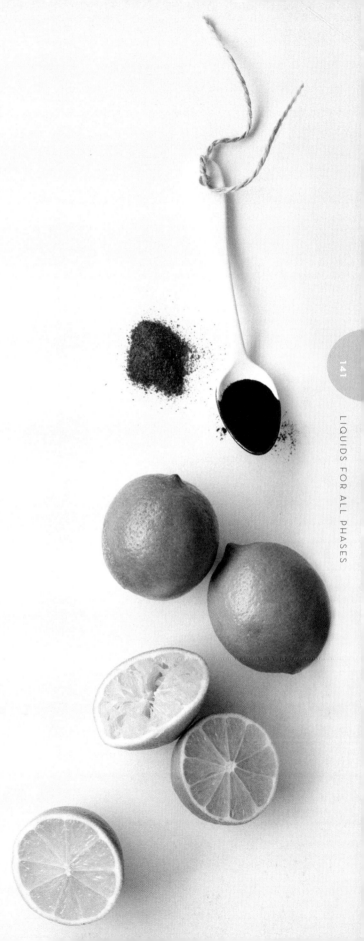

GO GREEN JUICE

Having a Go Green Juice every morning is the single most beneficial habit you can adopt to improve your health. It is not only wonderfully alkalising, but also provides you with a big dose of natural vitamins, minerals and amino acids to get you going for the day.

Including a tablespoon of essential fatty acid such as flaxseed oil or an omega-3 oil blend will mean you've taken your much-needed good oils for the day, as well as helping to maintain blood sugar levels and aid weight loss.

The Go Green Juice, as the name implies, is made up mainly of vegetables, not fruit. Only apples, pears, kiwifruits, pawpaw, berries, pineapples, lemons and limes should be used in the Go Green Juice mix, and mostly for taste purposes (although they also provide you with wonderful nutrients).

Choose dark green leafy vegetables such as kale, silverbeet, spinach, beet greens, rocket, watercress, chicory, comfrey or mustard greens as your base. Then add vegies such as beetroot, carrot, cabbage, celery or cucumber. And include alfalfa, coriander, parsley, mint, kelp, ginger or garlic for extra detoxifying powers.

After you have completed the program and are no longer having the other drinks, add 1 tablespoon of chia seeds or flaxseeds or linseed, sunflower and almond meal and 1 tablespoon of your chosen omega-3 oil to your daily Go Green Juice for your continuing fibre and essential fatty acid needs.

Amounts have not been included here as people's tastes vary. Play around with different combinations and amounts to work out what you prefer. Aim for 250–300 ml daily.

GO GREEN JUICE 1

Carrot
Celery
Cucumber
Green apple
Lemon juice
Parsley
Watercress

GO GREEN JUICE 3

Carrot
Coriander
Kale
Kiwifruit
Lime
Spinach

GO GREEN JUICE 2

Beetroot
Carrot
Celery
Cucumber
Garlic (optional)
Ginger
Lemon

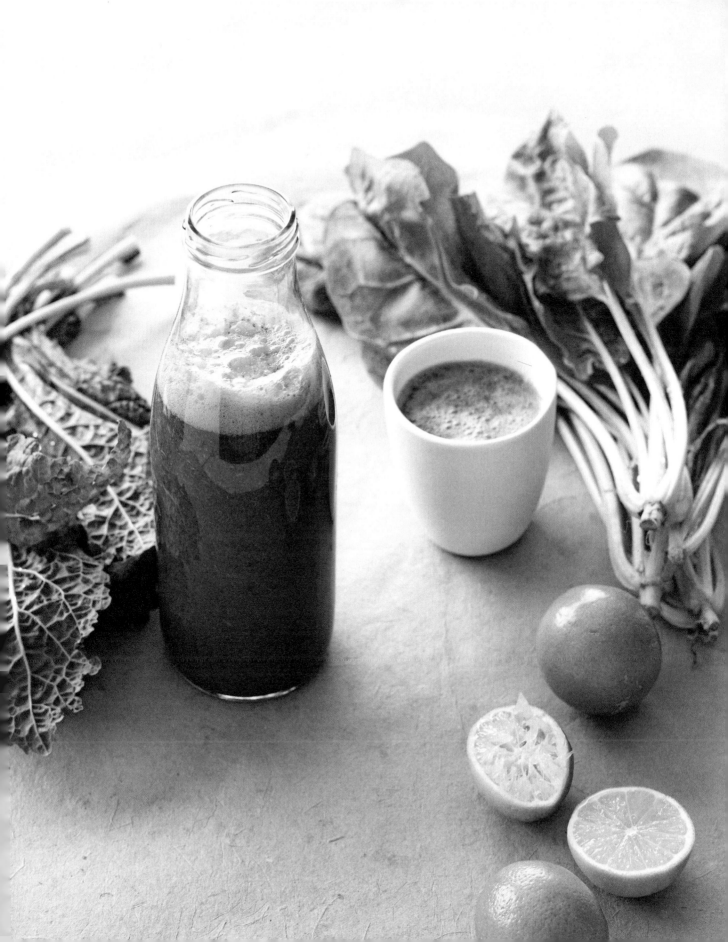

JUICES

ARISE & SHINE

A boost of vitamin C to kick-start your day.

SERVES 1

¼ pineapple, roughly chopped
100 g kale
2 kiwifruit, peeled and roughly chopped
1 lime, peeled

Juice and serve.

KICK-A-GERM JUICE

The quantities given here are approximate – you can use up to three lemons or five limes and up to four cloves of garlic if you like a stronger taste. Dried thyme can be substituted for fresh.

SERVES 1

1 lemon or 2 limes, skin on, chopped
2 cloves garlic, chopped
2 cm piece fresh ginger, peeled and chopped
½ teaspoon thyme leaves

Place all ingredients in a large jug, pour over 1 litre water and stir. Allow to stand for 10 minutes.

Strain a glassful at a time and drink throughout the day, topping up the jug with water as you go.

Each batch will last for 24 hours.

SORE HEAD

A great hangover cure.

SERVES 1

2 stalks celery, leaves left on
2 carrots
1 beetroot
1 bunch spinach
2 cm piece fresh ginger, peeled and chopped
1 clove garlic, peeled

Juice and serve.

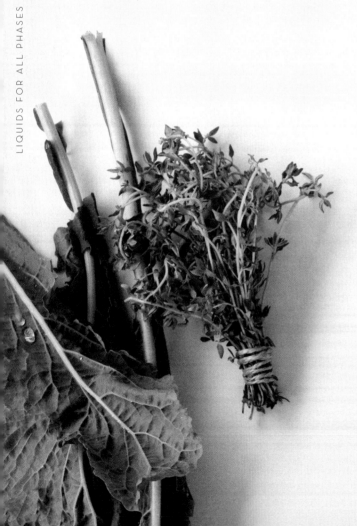

FACE LIFT

High in vitamins A, C, E and zinc for
a glowing complexion.

SERVES 1

1½ tomatoes
1 stalk celery, leaves left on
1 bunch spinach
3 carrots
¼ cup flat-leaf parsley leaves

Juice and serve.

DIGESTIVE DELIGHT

A super digestive cleanser. Also great
for reducing bloating.

SERVES 1

⅓ pineapple, chopped
50 g rocket
100 g coriander leaves
2 cm piece fresh ginger
80 g mint leaves
½ teaspoon fennel seeds

Juice, mix with 200 ml water and serve.

BLOOD CLEANSER

As the name suggests, also great for
a kidney and liver cleanse.

SERVES 1

1–2 green apples
2 stalks celery, leaves left on
350 g watercress
¼ cup flat-leaf parsley
2 beetroots
½ lemon

Juice and serve.

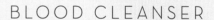
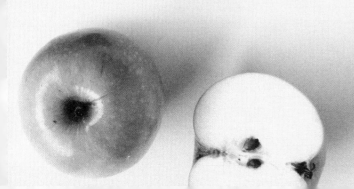

SMOOTHIES

POWER START

If this smoothie seems too thick, blend in a little more almond or rice milk.

SERVES 2

2 ripe medium bananas
75 g blueberries
1 tablespoon LSA (linseed, sunflower and almond mix)
2 eggs
1 small pawpaw, skin and seeds removed, roughly chopped
250 ml almond or rice milk
1 tablespoon raw honey or agave syrup

Blend all ingredients in a blender until creamy and serve.

NINJA SMOOTHIE

SERVES 2

1 green apple, cored, cut into chunks
1 pear, cored, cut into chunks
1 kiwifruit (skin on), ends cut off, quartered
1 bunch kale or watercress, washed, ends trimmed
250 ml rice, oat, soy, nut or seed milk

Place fruit in blender, then kale or watercress, pour over milk and blend until greens are completely liquefied and the mixture has a smooth consistency. Serve immediately.

CACAO-CASHEW SMOOTHIE

This to-die-for smoothie tastes so delicious and decadent, it's hard to believe it's a detox drink. It is meant to have a nutty consistency, ie quite bitty, but if you prefer a thinner consistency, blend in a little more water or milk.

SERVES 2

75 g cashews, soaked in water overnight
120 g fresh medjool dates, pitted
2 tablespoons raw cacao nibs
sea salt

Drain and rinse cashews and place in a blender along with dates, cacao powder and a pinch of sea salt. Add 500 ml water and blend until creamy. Serve immediately.

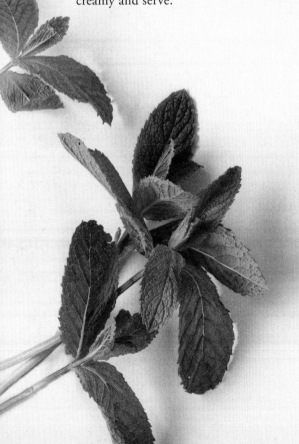

SUN SALUTE SMOOTHIE

SERVES 1

1–2 tablespoons sheep or goat's milk yoghurt
1 tablespoon LSA (linseed, sunflower seed and
    almond mix)
250 ml rice milk
handful of berries (raspberries, boysenberries,
    blueberries, Inca (or golden) berries,
    sumac or goji)
1 small banana
almond milk or water, for thinning (optional)

Blend all ingredients until creamy. If desired,
add a little almond milk or water for a
thinner consistency. Serve immediately.

DOWNWARD DOG SMOOTHIE

SERVES 1

250 ml rice, oat, soy, nut or seed milk, plus extra
    for thinning
1 small pawpaw
juice of ½ lime
2 cm piece fresh ginger, grated
1 tablespoon combination omega oil (such as Udo's
    3-6-9 blend)
handful ice cubes

Blend all ingredients in a blender until
creamy. Add a little more milk or water
as desired for a thinner consistency. Serve
immediately.

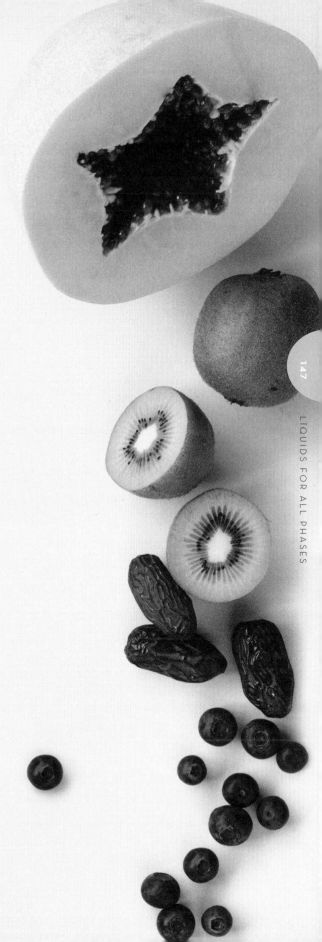

NUT & SEED MILKS

VANILLA HEMP MILK

Yes, hemp seed is from the cannabis plant, but it's not about to make you high! Hemp seeds are touted a superfood as they contain complete essential amino acids and essential fatty acids. Superfood or not, they are definitely nutritional powerhouses. You can purchase them in specialty health food shops or online.

MAKES 1.5 LITRES

45 g hulled hemp seeds
seeds from ½ vanilla pod
sea salt

Place hemp and vanilla seeds with 1.5 litres filtered water and a pinch of sea salt in a blender. Blend on high speed for 1–2 minutes until creamy.

For creamier milk, leave the pulp in; otherwise strain through a nut bag (also available in specialty health food shops) or muslin, squeezing out all of the liquid and discarding the pulp.

Store hemp milk in a glass bottle in the fridge for up to 4 days.

ENERGY DRINK >

As the name suggests, this drink gives you a real boost. You can use different spices such as ginger or chai spice mix.

SERVES 2

8 raw almonds
2 fresh medjool dates, pitted
4 cardamom pods
1 teaspoon fennel seeds
250 ml dairy-free milk

Soak all ingredients overnight in 250 ml water. Blend with milk and drink.

ALMOND MILK

If you prefer your milk a little sweet, add the medjool dates and vanilla. It will last 4 days if unsweetened, 2 days if sweetened.

MAKES 750 ML

160 g raw almonds
2 fresh medjool dates (optional), pitted
½ teaspoon pure vanilla extract (optional)
sea salt (optional)

Place almonds in a large bowl, cover with filtered water and leave to soak overnight. Drain and rinse, discarding soaking water. Place in a blender with 750 ml filtered water, dates, vanilla and salt if using.

Blend for 1–2 minutes or until very creamy. Strain through muslin, squeezing out all the liquid.

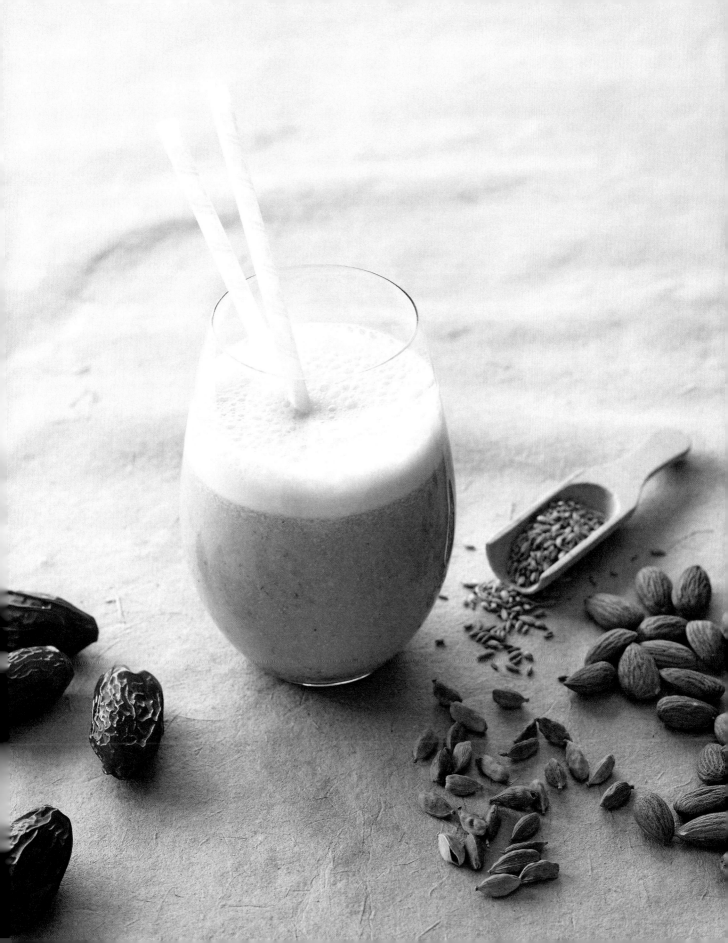

TEA

DETOXIFYING GINGER TEA

This tea draws toxins from the gastrointestinal tract, improves digestion
and strengthens your vital force.

1–2 teaspoons fresh grated ginger
¼ teaspoon ground fennel
¼ teaspoon ground cumin
¼ teaspoon ground coriander
¼ teaspoon ground cinnamon
natural sweetener such as raw honey, agave
   syrup or stevia, to taste (optional)

Add the spices to 1 litre water and bring to
the boil. Remove from heat, cover and allow
to steep for 5–10 minutes. Strain. The tea will
continue to get stronger the longer it steeps.
You can vary the amount of spice and the
mix of spices according to your taste. Add
sweetener of choice to taste, if preferred.

DEREK RIELLY, *magazine editor*

and cool dad to Jones and Garde

To keep up with my kids, I mentally shift from whatever work I've got going on to 'kids' time'. If you involve yourself completely in the moment, you'll love their company. If you're forever checking emails and messages or trying to read, you'll drive yourself nuts. I've also become deathly afraid of hangovers. Even at the very apex of an over-the-top night, the word 'kids' will flash into my brain around midnight and I'll pull back on the double vodkas or the tequila, scoop myself off the floor and dive into a taxi. Once I get home, I make sure I rehydrate with lots of water – a tip I learned from Saimaa.

To make sure my kids stay healthy, I'm careful not to project mainstream ideals of what constitutes a treat on to my little tigers. No kid needs Coke or the junk from vending machines. If you never buy it, it doesn't exist in their heads. It sure is a good feeling when a kid begs for an apple or a pear. Take your kids to the pool or beach instead giving them video games. Make them proud of their strength and their health, not their ability to manipulate their thumbs.

My top tip for staying healthy is: get outside. We live in such an awesome country where even the winters aren't that cold, so we have no excuse – move every chance you get. Run upstairs, run to your car, skip, swim at the beach. When it's raining, stretch in front of the TV or in the shower. Sing often and loudly. When you go out and liquor is doing its thing? Dance and don't stop – the mornings after are so much sweeter, hangover-wise. Health is everything. Money is pretty awesome, too, but don't sacrifice your vessel on the rocks pursuing it.

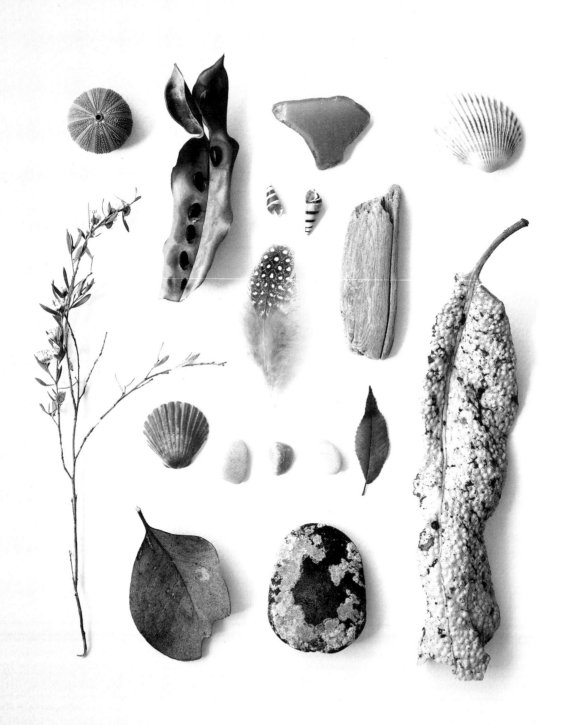

PART THREE

WHERE ARE YOU AT?

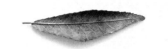

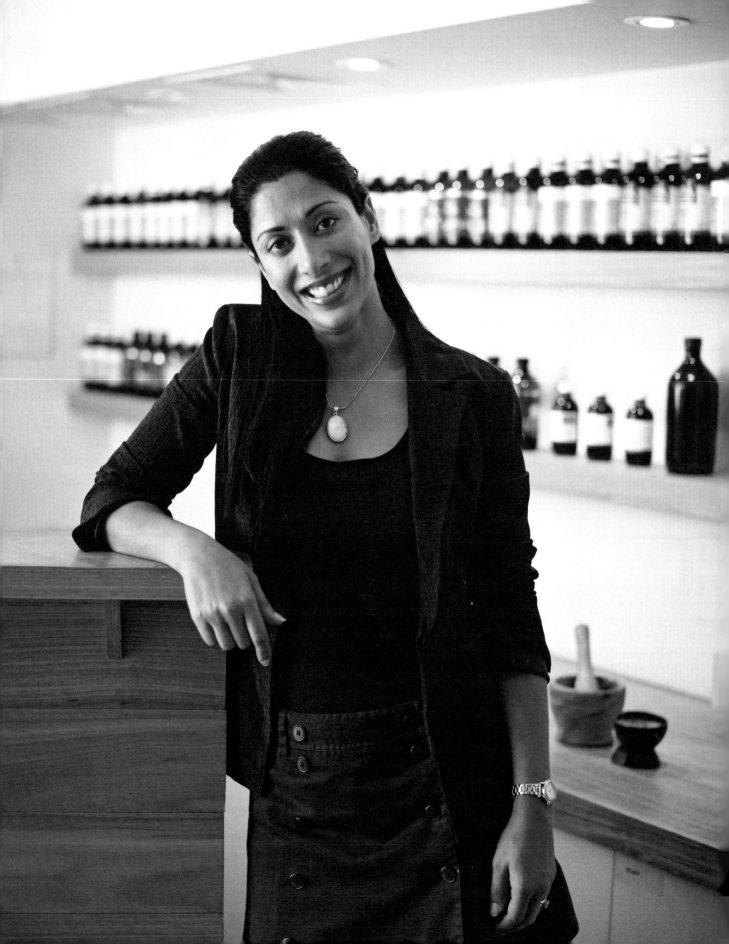

Well done you! You've completed the Aussie Body Diet detox and you're probably feeling a million bucks. Reflect on your journey and what it took to get you here. Check in with your goals to measure what you've achieved. Write down anything you've learnt about yourself. So, how does it feel to be optimally healthy, look and feel radiant, be more in control of your thoughts and striving to achieve your best?

One of the basic principles of the Aussie Body Diet is that life is ever-changing. It should never be stagnant. This part of the plan is all about maintenance; I'm going to arm you with knowledge and tools that are relevant to where you are in your life – and your true nature. We're going to move through different stages in life. When we're younger we tend to be more hedonistic, living for the moment, looking for instant gratification. This is completely OK. Some of us go through a phase where we're a little fanatical. When children come along, you can find your priorities change dramatically. When they leave the nest, your priorities change again. It's all part and parcel of growing up . . . and older. Then we all have our own issues, loves, interests, flaws, dreams . . . it's what makes us unique.

So use this section however you want to. There are no rules. Read it word-for-word and soak up more secrets, or keep it as a handy reference. Come back to the book as you move through different stages in your life. Most importantly, allow yourself to be flexible and adaptable; accommodate the ebb and flow of life.

1
THE HEDONIST

'Our deepest fear is not that we are
inadequate. Our deepest fear is that we are
powerful beyond measure.'

— Nelson Mandela

We've all been hedonistic at some point in our lives. If you haven't, it's bound to happen. From enjoying gourmet dinners every night to backpacking through Europe on a diet of beer and Pringles, the Hedonist is in constant pursuit of pleasure and instant gratification. It's good to do what feels good. It can be healthy. You can't be expected to practise restraint all the time – it's not realistic. Rigidity isn't good for your mental or physical wellbeing. And natural medicine experts believe rigidity causes acidity in our bodies. As long as you're not harming yourself, appreciate the hedonistic phase.

If you're in it right now, why are you reading this book? Did someone give it to you as a hint? Are you reading it because you want to change? Are you overweight, lethargic or depressed? Do you want to toss the cigarettes? Cut back on the grog? Give up recreational drugs? Do you want to balance a heady lifestyle with good, stabilising habits? My hope is that no matter what your situation, you'll find some solutions here.

If you've completed the detox, reap the rewards by taking yourself out to your favourite restaurant, bar or club and enjoy the smokin' hot new you (accompanied by wolf whistles, double-takes and all). You now have a blank canvas to work with and know that you can still enjoy yourself by living with Aussie Body Diet principles. If you haven't, maybe you've realised by now that you can still be a hedonist but you'll feel much, much better if you did the 14-day detox now and again. Cleansing your body from time to time is the best way to get perspective and eliminate harmful toxins. It's OK to revert to your hedonistic ways after the 14-day detox program. Optimal health is a work in progress. And if you are truly wanting to get over a substance addiction, then I believe you need to alkalise your body and commit to the 14-day program. It will help you to get rid of addiction on a cellular level and strengthen your mind so you can clearly see the addiction for what it is.

Even if you keep up the decadence after the program, I guarantee you'll party more wisely with each detox under your belt. Not because you're suffering, but because it will start to feel like the right thing. I've seen it many times. Your body will love you because you are providing yourself with alkalising nutrients, which in turn combats the harmful effects of having too much acidity in the body (unfortunately a product of extravagance).

If you do nothing else after the program but continue to hydrate (three litres of filtered water daily) and make the Go Green Juice most mornings (add one tablespoon of chia seeds or flaxseed, plus one tablespoon of good oil), then you've already done wonders for your body. Oh, and don't mix paracetamol with alcohol, even when you feel your head might explode. Your liver will hate you.

So enjoy where you're at and don't feel guilty – guilt is a waste of time. Laugh a lot, get up before noon occasionally, soak up some sunshine and surround yourself with nature. The Irish have a saying: 'A good laugh and a long sleep are the best cures in the doctor's book.' And they should know.

TIPS FOR THE HEDONIST

1. Don't see anything as good or bad for you.

2. Don't allow yourself to say, 'I can't'. Even when you're hungover.

3. Hydrate, hydrate and hydrate some more. It will get rid of toxins and also curb hunger.

4. Practise food-combining at dinner time to speed up digestion before sleep.

5. Shoot for regular meal times: your circadian rhythm craves routine.

6. When eating out, always have a salad as an entree to kick-start digestion.

7. Be mindful of every mouthful: think of food as fuel for the body and chew it well.

8. On big nights out, have one or two beers or glasses of wine, then move on to spirits, which contain the least amount of yeast. Mix spirits with fresh lime and soda instead of sugary mixers.

9. Get seven to eight hours' sleep every night. Sleep deprivation is linked to weight gain as it can result in a rise in cortisol, which is appetite-inducing. Anything less than this causes you to crave sugary and fattening foods.

10. If you're quitting an addiction, be firm in your decision and stick to it. Use supplements, the NET diary on p 199 and therapies as aids. Seek counselling if you need to. Don't second-guess yourself. Instead, keep yourself occupied with other activities and know that the craving *always* goes.

FACTS ABOUT FAT

The benefits of essential fatty acids are widely known and accepted. Even doctors prescribe omega-rich foods and supplements. Why? Because your body can't manufacture its own essential fatty acids and they're a vital part of all cell membranes. They help the body absorb fat-soluble vitamins A, D, E and K. The brain is 60 per cent fat and research suggests getting enough essential fatty acids could help thwart depression. Essential fatty acids are a back-up source of energy, form a vital part of the membrane of every cell in your body and make up the protective layer that surrounds our vital organs such as the liver, brain and heart. Good oils also play a vital role in hormone and immune function.

Essential fatty acids are divided into omega 3, omega 6 and 9. Good sources of omega 3 include flaxseed, mustard seeds, walnuts, tofu, cod liver oil and oily fish (tuna, salmon, cod, trout, mackerel, sardines and herrings). Sources of omega 6 include lecithin, sunflower oil, corn, safflower, sesame, hemp, chia seed, pumpkin, evening primrose and borage oil. Omegas 9s are non-essential, but are still considered 'good' oils, and include mono-unsaturated fats such as olive oil.

These 'good' fats are brimming with benefits. Omega 3 fats, in particular, lower blood pressure and levels of bad cholesterol (triglycerides), while boosting levels of good cholesterol (HDL) and, in turn, cut your risk of heart disease, stroke and cancer. They reduce inflammation, improve bone density – which protects against osteoporosis – and can alleviate PMS and period pain. They even aid in weight loss.

The saturated fats in animal meat and dairy products are considered the 'baddies' in terms of fats. While omega fatty acids guard against disease, too much saturated fat has been linked to heart disease and cancer. But not all saturated fats are created equal. Virgin coconut oil is high in saturated fat but it's a type called lauric acid, which is considered less harmful. In fact, lauric acid can increase levels of helpful HDL cholesterol in the blood, which is good for your ticker.

The undeniable villains of the fat world are transfats – polyunsaturated oils that have been hydrogenated, or converted into a solid form.

They're most often used in processed foods like margarine, baked goods and biscuits, as they're cheap, stable and extend shelf life. Transfats lower levels of good HDL cholesterol and bump up bad cholesterol, and high intake leads to obesity. In a six-year study, monkeys who were fed transfats gained seven per cent of their body weight, compared with 1.7 per cent in the primates who ate healthy, monounsaturated fats. Poor monkeys!

A word on the good oils: only consume cold-pressed, unrefined oil (with olive oil, look for 'extra virgin'). And don't overheat: oils can oxidise, creating free radicals – chemicals that have been linked to cancer. For cooking purposes, olive oil, coconut oil, sesame oil, ghee and butter are safe to use.

After you've completed the 14-day program, it's still a great idea to put one tablespoon of chia seeds and one tablespoon of liquid EFA such as Udo's 3-6-9 Oil Blend, or flaxseed or hemp seed oil into your Go Green Juice to help meet your daily EFA needs.

THE POWER OF HABIT

It's human nature to form habits. Whether they're good or bad, the old adage says it takes three weeks to make or break a habit. So, do anything consistently for 21 days and it becomes second nature – as automatic as brushing teeth, checking your phone or cleaning your plate. Or quit something for 21 days – cigarettes, trashy TV, needing something sweet after every meal– and you'll retrain your brain to knock that habit for good. Sure, you might relapse. But that's also part of human nature, part of the ebb and flow of life. When you're ready, get back on the horse!

As unconscious as these habits feel, you are in control of your behaviour. The Aussie Body

Diet is not about wagons; I'm not going to wave my finger at you for falling off (in fact I'm going to commend you for trying). It's about cleansing the body so you can enjoy the occasional big night out or lazy Sunday DVD marathon armed with some serious snackage. In a nutshell, the Aussie Body diet and detox plan is about tipping the scale so that healthier options take precedence over unhealthier ones – rather than the other way around!

JUST MOVE

As we discussed in Chapter Four (Movement), exercise doesn't need to be a chore. You should enjoy it, so find an activity that inspires you. Make it a priority. Just move your body – and not just on the dance floor. When you don't exercise often, you're more susceptible to injuries and pain. If you suddenly go hard, you could hurt yourself or be too sore to get up off the couch. Cue the downward spiral! Go easy and challenge yourself incrementally. Your patience will be rewarded. Remember, exercise oxygenates the blood, massages your internal organs and gets your body firing on all cylinders. It slows down the internal and external effects of the ageing process.

You're a social person, right? Instead of meeting at the pub, coerce your friends into a soccer match or coastal walk. Set yourself mini-challenges to keep things interesting. If you're walking or running, stop at intervals and work your big muscle groups with squats, lunges, push-ups, triceps dips and abdominal work. That's all it takes to create beautiful contours in your body. If you need a push, enlist a personal trainer. It doesn't mean forking out wads of cash for life; personal trainers can help you get started, design a program and coach you in proper form. Hey, mix socialising and personal training sessions while saving moolah by getting a group together. Whatever you choose, make the commitment to move more and often. Remember, consistency is the key.

EAT FRESH

Packaged food is often cooked at very high temperatures or loaded up with preservatives and additives. The process can require a lot of water and natural resources – think of all that plastic – so it's more costly to our environment. Then there are the emissions from transporting food in trucks all over the country. Natural medicine experts believe that processed foods are acid-forming and harder for our bodies to digest than whole foods. They can be filled with unnecessary toxins and can be harmful to our health. Choosing food that's as close as possible to its original, whole form is one of the Aussie Body Diet's secret lifestyle principles and one of the best habits you can adopt. I guarantee it will improve digestion and vitality – and cut back on medical bills.

RUSS AYRES, *NLP master business coach*

As a self-confessed workaholic and loving what I do, I didn't notice how little attention I was paying to my own wellbeing. Previously I always enjoyed running and weight training, but that had really taken a back seat until I thought I should get fit again.

I heard about Saimaa's work through a celebrity client of hers who lives here in London. The next opportunity I had, I went to see this 'witch doctor' who came so highly recommended.

Consulting with Saimaa revealed that my diet was quite poor and my cellular age was over fifty! Still, I thought will alone should be all I needed to regain my fitness level; this proved incorrect.

I adopted Saimaa's detox program and within days I noticed a change in my energy levels. On day nine that I woke up after a very restful sleep and realised I actually wanted to go to the gym. So I got my gear on and worked out. Now I was compelled to exercise pretty much every day, and soon I was feeling fantastic with a cellular age of 31 (I'm 38) and a body fat percentage of 12 per cent (prior to the detox I'm embarrassed to say it was 36 per cent).

The changes to my body were visually obvious after the first week of the program, and I was far more productive at work. I found I was able to make decisions more efficiently and my mood stabilised. It was only on reflection that I realised just how stressed I had been before.

Maintenance is easy: I simply follow the rule of eighteen meals per week of high-quality nutrition, and three meals of whatever I like.

Overall, I was shocked at just how quickly my body repaid me for detoxing. I owe it to Saimaa but she always tells me it's all me!

DAMIAN WALSHE-HOWLING, *actor, writer, director*

The Aussie Body 14-day diet has become a yearly ritual for me over the past eight years. The power of detoxification became blindingly clear during my first cleanse many years ago. Not only did my physical health improve immensely but I experienced a calm and clarity that had been evasive up to that point, due to all the excesses in my lifestyle. My favourite saying is 'Everything in moderation, including moderation itself.' Health and detoxification have as much to do with following your own intuitive wisdom as they do with systems of diet and exercise.

Experiencing the health that comes from detoxifying has encouraged me to pursue a healthier lifestyle overall; however at times I also need to let loose, because occasional indulgence is not only fun but essential to a balanced life. Health for me is an energised state of flow in which I am truly able to not only listen but also to follow the ever-changing needs of my daily experience. Some days that means rest and extra sleep, others it means pushing myself on many levels, but most of all it means existing in harmony with those around me and my environment.

2
THE FAT FIGHTER

'Anything is achievable as long as your
commitment is constant and consistent.'

— Anthony Robbins

Magazine covers are littered with weight-loss headlines, slimmers have become reality TV stars and health-food companies can make meal replacement bars look like chocolate. Weight-loss advice is everywhere, yet reaching a happy, healthy weight is still a struggle for so many. But it's very possible. Whether you want to completely overhaul your body or just lose that last couple of kilos, slow, sustainable weight loss is within your reach. My patients have found that when they alkalise their bodies, everything works as it should – optimally.

Hopefully you've completed the detox – nice work – and your body's a clean slate. It's time to commit to no fad diets. The reason fad diets don't work is because they drastically restrict your food intake. Who wants a milkshake for lunch . . . for the rest of their life? Or to worry about the carbs in a carrot? Or to actually think avocados are bad for you? A fad diet is a band-aid solution and not sustainable. Extreme kilojoule restriction can trigger the 'feast or famine' response, where the body suspects it's entering a phase of starvation, slows the metabolism and clings to fat reserves. Go on enough diets and you'll screw up your metabolism for life, so when you do eat normally, you'll stack on the kilos. Hunger pangs can lead to binges. Restricting your food intake also reduces lean muscle mass, and as we now know muscle burns through energy even when you're not exercising. Less muscle: more fat.

My biggest beef with short-term fad diets: they encourage a negative preoccupation with food. Dieters see foods as 'good' or 'bad'. It messes with your head! A diet should be a long-term, sustainable plan that nourishes you. After all, as I've said before, food is *meant* to be enjoyed.

Reaching and maintaining your happy weight is important to your health. It shouldn't be about sizes, attracting the opposite sex or having an insanely great body (though the latter is a nice bonus). Unfortunately, being overweight or obese increases the risk of heart disease, type 2 diabetes, cancer, high blood pressure, sleep apnoea, osteoarthritis, depression and reproductive obstacles. Make the prevention of serious diseases your motivation, rather than what you see in the mirror.

HEALTHY TIPS FOR LOSING WEIGHT

1. Drink three litres of water, minimum, per day. Mix it up with herbal teas.

2. Increase your intake of fibre with vegetables, wholegrains, legumes, nuts, seeds and psyllium husks. Fibre is filling and will prevent you from overeating. It also lowers cholesterol.

3. Aim for one serve of protein with every meal to stabilise blood sugar levels. Aim for 0.8 grams of protein for every kilogram of body weight.

4. Consume complex carbohydrates (grains) during the day, when you're more active. Aim for only *one* grain meal per day.

5. Eat dinner early – at least three hours before sleeping, so you won't disrupt your circadian rhythm, which in turn affects your appetite hormones.

6. Take a few deep breaths before starting your meal to calm the nervous system and aid digestion. When we're stressed, the body increases cortisol, which promotes fat storage.

7. Slow down and chew properly; this gives your body time to recognise when it's full.

8. Don't skip meals – doing so may lead to overeating or bingeing later on.

9. Always check the labels of processed foods, as they usually contain sugars and additives. Sugar's a major contributor to obesity and type 2 diabetes.

10. Get enough sleep to stimulate the appetite-suppressing hormone, leptin, and to lower levels of the appetite-promoting hormone ghrelin.

THERE'S NOTHING SWEET ABOUT SUGAR

The increasing rate of type 2 diabetes and obesity is largely thanks to our over-consumption of sugar, which is often hidden in processed foods from instant soups to cereal. Any sugar (carbohydrates) from food that you don't immediately use gets stored as fat. And being overweight – especially if you're an 'apple' shape – is a big risk factor for type 2 diabetes.

In healthy people, insulin is a hormone produced by the pancreas that collects glucose from the blood and delivers it to the cells of the body for energy. At the same time, insulin stops the liver from producing more glucose.

In people with type 2 diabetes – usually occurring in adulthood, thanks to a poor diet and lack of exercise – not enough insulin is made, which means more glucose circulates through the blood instead of reaching the muscles where it's needed. Then excess sugar becomes a really, really big problem.

Moreover, sugar increases the production of a type of free radical called 'advanced glycation end products', when a sugar molecule binds to a protein or lipid. These contribute to inflammation, atherosclerosis, Alzheimer's disease and somewhat less seriously, wrinkles. Sugar also impairs the construction of collagen, leading to reduced skin elasticity.

And you don't need to be a food scientist to know that eating sugar promotes mood swings and irritability. Sure, inhaling a bag of M&Ms will make you feel good for half an hour. But what goes up must come down.

Refined sugar should be avoided at all costs – it is completely devoid of nutrients. Sugar comes in many forms. When you're looking at labels, anything ending in 'ose' is a sugar: glucose, sucrose, fructose. Maltodextrin, corn syrup and molasses are also varieties of sugar. Steer clear of artificial sweeteners; studies show they also contribute to obesity, as you get a hit of sweetness without the satiety. They only make your cravings worse.

It's easy to become addicted to sugar. When any substance affects us on a cellular level, if we don't consume that substance, it causes us to experience cravings. The hard part is quitting. If you've followed the 14-day diet, you've already kicked sugar's butt. If not, it's time to ban the white stuff. At first, the cravings might drive you mad, but in less than two weeks, I promise you'll be able to sit in front of the most delectable dessert and resist. Yes, even macarons.

Remember natural medicine experts believe that sugar affects the pH of our blood, which in turn changes our palate to be more acidic. That is why the more sugar you have, the more you crave. Once you've forgotten what refined sugar tastes like, you'll find that carrots and beetroot are super-sweet. Even rice tastes sweet. Try it!

ATTITUDE IS ALL

When it comes to weight loss, a positive attitude will get you over the line. *Not* gimmicks. You need to find inspiration in nutritious food and the motivation to exercise (hint: it's already within you). You need the right attitude before you can adopt and stick to positive, healthy habits.

As we discussed in Chapter Five (Positive Outlook), your mind is a powerful tool. It's your mind that will help you achieve your very best; no-one else can do it for you. Learn to recognise your negative thinking patterns

and replace them with positive affirmations. Do this often enough and your brain will start seeing those affirmations as a reality. A wonderful self-fulfilling prophecy!

FAD-FREE WEIGHT LOSS

If you're serious about fighting the flab (and have the all-clear from your health practitioner), shoot for high-intensity cardiovascular exercise for 45 minutes, at least five times per week. Jogging, cycling, dancing, boxing, skipping or the cross trainer are my picks. If you're more of a walker, punish the pavement and try to break a sweat. Fartlek training – a funny name for interval training – is gold. You alternate between two- to five-minute bursts of high-intensity exercise and recovery breaks of slower or low-intensity work.

Whatever you do, strive to reach 80 per cent of your maximum heart rate and keep it up – you should be puffing. I believe first thing in the morning, before breakfast, is the optimal time for fat burning. Because you've fasted overnight, your body's more likely to churn through stored carbohydrates and fat rather than any carbs from brekkie or lunch. Try to include at least one yoga session per week to boost flexibility, strengthen your core and reduce injuries, on top of your post-workout stretches.

SUPPORTIVE SUPPLEMENTS

Here's a short list of natural supplements that may aid your weight-loss efforts. It's much better for the environment to use natural, biodegradable preparations rather than synthetic and prescription medications. See a naturopath for the best dosages for your individual needs.

- Brindleberry (*Garcinia cambogia*): known to inhibit the synthesis of lipids, lower 'bad' cholesterol (LGL and triglycerides) and inhibit the storing of kilojoules as body fat.

- Cacao (*Theobroma cacao*): the antioxidants and methylxanthines in cacao can help reduce your appetite and get your eating behaviours under control. They also work in a similar way to some antidepressants, inhibiting serotonin reuptake in the brain, which can make you feel good and thus help prevent 'emotional eating'.

- Caralluma (*Caralluma fimbriata*): an appetite suppressant that works on the hunger sensory mechanism of the hypothalamus (in your brain). Also enhances endurance and increases fat metabolism.

- Chilli and cayenne pepper (*Capsicum annuum, minimum or fastigiatum*): thermogenic (warming) herbs that stimulate the circulatory system and boost metabolism. They also increase the body's ability to utilise fat stores.

- Chromium: this essential mineral can't be made by the body but it's necessary for proper carbohydrate, fat and protein metabolism, and according to research it may improve insulin sensitivity and thus help ward off type 2 diabetes.

- Green tea (*Camellia sinensis*): high in antioxidants and it increases leptin, which suppresses appetite. The antioxidant epigallocatechin-3-0-gallate (EGCG) in green tea has warming effects.

- Gymnema (*Gymnema sylvestre*): widely used by naturopaths to treat obesity and diabetes. Regulates blood sugar, suppresses appetite and is an anaesthetic on the sweet-receptive taste buds.

- L-carnitine: an amino acid that helps convert fat into usable energy. Food sources include asparagus, avocado, beef, lamb, chicken, fish and tempeh.

- Yacon: a root vegetable from South America; its sweetness comes from inulin (a fibre, not to be confused with insulin). Helps manage cholesterol, triglyceride and blood sugar levels.

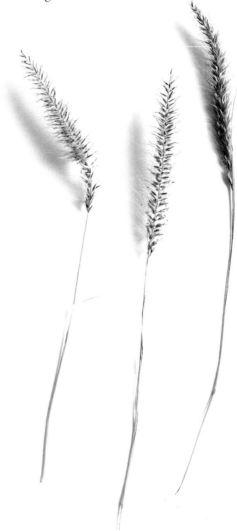

LORRAINE WILSON, *store owner*

I am a 50-year-old woman, married with three grown-up children. I work at least 55 hours a week in a general store my husband and I have owned for five years.

Overall I felt my health was OK before detox. I basically followed the same routine year in, year out: get up early 6 days a week, work hard, walk or jog with the dog every day, and reward myself later in the evening with two or three glasses of wine. However, I felt tired most of the time and put it down to hard work. I embarked on the detox program with doubts in my mind – I wasn't sure I was actually capable of changing my habits.

Day 1 was a bit tricky due to vast quantities of alcohol consumed the previous night with friends. I was determined not to break the detox on the very first day and got through unscathed, happy to go to bed without a nightcap!

Day 2 kicked in and I was on track. I had bought all the allowable foods and made dinner and lunches for the next few days. This made it easier, especially for work and late evenings. Food was on my mind but because of the healthy snacks, I never went hungry. By 5 p.m. I noticed slight headaches but they weren't too bad. I was already used to exercising every day, so that wasn't a problem.

From Day 3, I began to notice small changes in my appearance. The wrinkles had lessened and my bloated menopausal middle was feeling a little less oversized. Darby (my husband) even

commented that my face looked younger and a couple of his friends had commented on how well I looked. With this sort of praise, I wanted to see how I'd look and feel at the end of the detox period.

Day 6 onwards was much easier: drinking water became a habit, food was enjoyable, and the lack of caffeine and alcohol in my life barely entered my thoughts – until some friends invited us for lunch. I warned them I was likely to be a bore and make a lame excuse to leave early as I would be the 'sober' one. To my surprise we stayed for four hours, and it was thoroughly enjoyable without alcohol.

Towards the end of the program, I felt my brain had been reset and I'd broken all my bad habits. Nothing was missing from my life; I actually felt in control. The icing on the cake was pulling on jeans that do up easily – and no muffin top! Customers at our shop have since asked for a copy of Saimaa's detox plan. I think they realised that if I can do it with my busy schedule, they can too.

As Saimaa suggested, I began with the 14-day gentle detox, followed by one week of maintenance, then the 14-day advanced detox, one week of maintenance, then back to the 14-day detox, doing three rounds in total.

It has been six months since I completed Saimaa's program. To date, I have lost 22 kilos, I look ten years younger, and I feel as good as I did in my twenties.

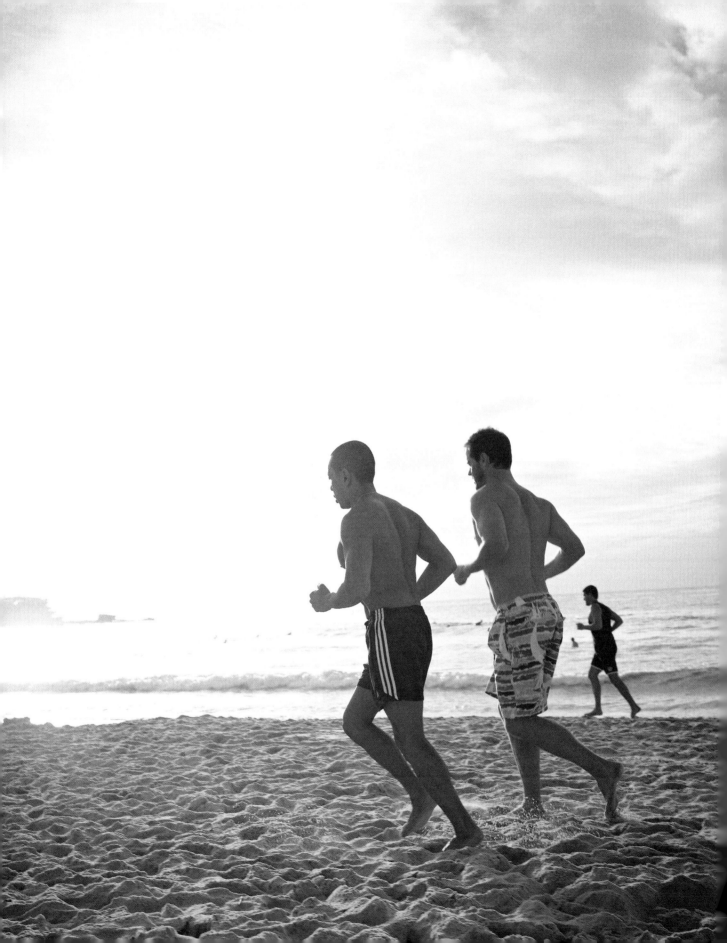

3
THE ATHLETE

'I know of no more encouraging fact than the
unquestionable ability of man to elevate his
life by a conscious endeavour.'

— Henry David Thoreau

Naturopaths, nutritionists and doctors love treating athletes and fitness freaks. You're so easy to work with! If you're an athlete (or want to be), you know your body is a temple and nourishing it with good, clean fuel will get you to peak condition. You know that diet is the ultimate performance-enhancing drug. And it's totally legal. In this chapter, I'm simply tweaking your good lifestyle habits so you can be on top of your game.

Improve your . . . strength. To build muscle, you need to feed it correctly. Party pies and hot chips won't get you to the Olympics. Avoid processed food and refined sugar; shoot for 100 per cent whole foods. A muscle-building diet should comprise 30 to 50 per cent protein, 20 to 50 per cent carbohydrates and 20 to 40 per cent fat (essential fatty acids). Different ratios will suit different athletes, so experiment to find the ratios that work best for you. If needed, consult with a naturopath or nutritionist. You need five to six small meals a day, to get enough kilojoules while keeping your blood sugars under control. Every meal should include some protein, as protein supplies the building blocks for muscle. Keep up your NET diary (see p 199).

Providing your body with the materials it needs to build muscle is only one part of increasing strength. A resistance training program is imperative for building muscle mass. Your workout should concentrate on compound weight-lifting exercises, which use multiple muscle groups, like the squat or bench press. Move weights that allow you to complete six to 12 repetitions per set, and two to three sets per exercise. Try to either increase the amount of weight lifted or the reps completed with each session. Don't go overboard with your strength training: two to three intense, one-hour workouts per week should do the trick. Leave a day in between working different muscle groups, as muscle fibres tear when you lift challenging weights. As the fibres rest and repair, the muscle becomes stronger.

Improve your . . . speed. To increase speed, you have to program your mind and body by training your fast-twitch muscle fibres. These determine how quickly your muscles react and contract; they are great for quick, powerful movements like jumping or sprinting. Because they use up loads of energy, fast-twitch fibres tire easily. Repetition is the best way to hone your fast-twitch muscle. Look at boxers: they'll go through endless rounds of hitting pads and the speedball, so when they're finally in the ring, they don't need to think about evading punches or blocking upper-cuts. It's an unconscious movement coming from fast-twitch muscle fibres that allows them to duck and weave in a flash.

Improve your . . . endurance. This is really important for peak performance: there's nothing worse than getting halfway through an event and finding you've no fuel left in the tank.

This is where slow-twitch muscle fibres do their stuff. They're rich in blood vessels so there's a constant supply of oxygen, meaning you can go harder for longer (but they don't boast the explosive power of fast-twitch fibres). Train your slow-twitch muscles with longer, aerobic exercise sessions rather than lose-your-breath anaerobic workouts. Remember, endurance is 90 per cent mental, as it's our minds that tell us to stop, to keep going, to go faster or to collapse into the foetal position! It's not always the body just 'conking out'. But obviously, it is helpful if we train our bodies to sustain a higher level of exertion over a longer period of time.

PEAK PERFORMANCE

1 Create a burning desire to succeed: watch other sportspeople for motivation.

2 Commit to a goal or an endpoint so you have clear direction.

3 Be adaptable – training doesn't always happen the way we'd like. Adjust and take responsibility for your outcome.

4 Visualise yourself reaching your goal in detail. Picture yourself sprinting over a finishing line, imagine the sound of crowds cheering, feel the weight of a trophy in your hand.

5 Muscles respond best when you change your routine, so vary your work-outs.

6 Be aware of your breath; diaphragm breathing allows more oxygen to circulate and helps you get rid of lactic acid, which causes muscle fatigue.

7 Work on your flexibility with yoga and stretching to reduce the risk of injuries. It's vital for peak performance.

8 Work on your balance – don't just train to your strongest side. Balance kinetic energy for a stronger body.

9 Recovery time is essential; take one day off per week. Rest allows muscles to release metabolic acids and give them the chance to grow without injury. Overtraining can lead to fatigue, burnout, depression and low immunity.

10 Detox regularly so your body isn't burdened with mopping up toxins. My athlete clients have found that the key to consistent performance is taking time to clean elimination channels and alkalise their bodies.

A GUIDE TO PROTEIN

Protein is necessary for the growth, repair and development of muscle – and to perform almost every activity in the body. Protein is broken down into amino acids, which are like the Swiss Army knife of nutrients (really, really useful). Amino acids build muscle, tendons and ligaments, make hormones and enzymes, and synthesise neurotransmitters, which control mood. Our bodies are capable of making some amino acids (called non-essential); however, some can only come from food (essential). Complete proteins contain all the essential amino acids. The best sources are eggs, meat, dairy products and soy bean products such as tofu.

Protein also helps regulate blood sugar levels by slowing down the digestion of carbohydrates and sugars. Stabilising blood sugar levels ensures a regular supply of energy, minimising fatigue and cravings.

SOURCES OF PROTEIN

- Animal sources: red meat, white meat, fish
- Dairy: milk, yoghurt, cheese
- Eggs
- Nuts and seeds: particularly chia, linseed, sunflower seeds and almonds
- Cruciferous vegies such as brussels sprouts and broccoli
- Grains: barley, corn, rye, millet, buckwheat, oats, amaranth, quinoa, wild rice, burghul
- Legumes: adzuki beans, dry peas, lentils, soy beans, kidney beans, black beans, baked beans, chickpeas
- Nori (seaweed) sheets, spirulina and micro-algae such as chlorella and marine phytoplankton
- Fermented foods: tofu, sourdough bread, tempeh, natto, kefir

CALCULATE YOUR PROTEIN INTAKE

Athletes need to aim for 1–1.2 g of protein per kilogram of body weight per day – so for example, if you weigh 75 kg, you'd need 90 g of protein a day. See the table on p 197 to help you ensure you're getting your dose. (All weights are cooked weights.)

FOCUS

Great athletes are very determined, focused and ambitious. They've harnessed the power of mind control. Athletes are disciplined and motivated not because they're wired differently, but because they've cultivated their minds to become physically and mentally tough. They weren't born that way. Athletes learn to withstand pain and choose not to listen to the negative voices inside their heads telling them 'You can't do it', or 'Can't we just have a little lie-down now?' Elite athletes see fear, pain and negativity as challenges to overcome and opportunities to transform themselves. This ability is in each and every one of us. As you think, so you are.

CORE WORK

A strong core is the foundation of fitness. It makes us stable and helps us to move easily. It helps us to correct our posture, reducing risk of injuries and back pain.

Our core is where our balance comes from and, in Oriental medicine, is where our 'chi' or energy centre in the body sits. The power in any big movement actually comes from our core, as using the body correctly involves the big muscle groups and the energy generated by our torsos.

FITNESS-BOOSTERS

- Adaptogenic herbs are traditionally used to increase the body's resistance to stress, producing a defensive response to stressors and allowing the body to increase exertion. Athletes are often prescribed Korean and Siberian ginseng, withania (aka ashwagandha), neem, licorice, astragalus, rhodiola and tribulus.

- Camu camu comes from the Amazonian rainforest and is known for its unusually high vitamin C content, which makes it a potent antioxidant that combats free radical damage from strenuous training. Other types of berries such as goji, Inca berries, sumac, acerola and acai are beneficial too.

- Chia and hemp seeds are a complete protein containing all amino acids, as well as essential fatty acids and minerals such as magnesium.

- Coconut water is loved by athletes for its super-hydrating qualities. It's loaded with calcium, potassium and magnesium, zinc, selenium, iodine, sulfur, manganese, boron, molybdenum, ascorbic acid and B-group vitamins – making it a fantastic electrolyte drink that is low in sugar.

- Coenzyme Q_{10}, also known as CoQ_{10} and 'ubiquinones', generates energy in the mitochondria of your cells. A CoQ_{10} supplement enhances energy production, and also functions as an antioxidant for the heart.

- Creatine can speed up the generation of adenosine triphosphate (ATP), which delivers much-needed energy to muscle cells, helping you to lift more weight and develop your muscles more quickly.

- Glutamine helps your muscles to repair and rebuild after training, meaning a faster recovery.

- Magnesium promotes nerve and muscle function, and bumper bone health. It's linked with reduced risk of diabetes, heart disease and osteoporosis. Magnesium promotes nerve and muscle relaxation, amongst other benefits, and is one of the important micro-nutrients for building healthy muscle tissue.

- Raw maca powder has a longstanding reputation as a strength and stamina booster. It also is known as a superfood for its complete vitamin and mineral content and can increase energy and endurance through oxygenating the blood.

| CASE STUDY |

TAJ BURROW, *pro surfer*

I grew up in a remote town in WA's south west surrounded by great surf. There was not much else to do apart from surfing, plus my parents were mad about surfing, so I guess you could say I had no choice about becoming a pro surfer – it was inevitable!

When I'm in training mode, my daily routine is basically: surf, train, stretch, hydrate and eat really good food. We do a lot of surf-specific exercises which focus on strength, balance and speed. We also do postural work to make sure my body is in alignment, which is great for injury prevention and focus on squatting, lunging, twisting, pulling, pushing and bending, as well as mixing it all up and keeping it fun. To recover, I stretch, play tennis, sleep and have massages.

Following Saimaa's guidelines, I eat a high-protein diet, organic when possible and stay away from processed foods and drinks. I drink only good-quality filtered water and lots of it.

In the down time between training and events, I'm guilty of being a couch potato – I love just relaxing in my own home because it's so rare.

For optimum fitness, besides the actual training, I think correct breathing, stretching, hydrating and believing in the exercise you're doing is very important.

The best Aussie lifestyle secret is 100 per cent the beach! Spending time at the beach and in the ocean makes everyone so much happier and healthier.

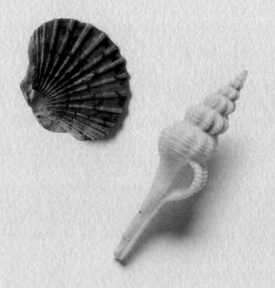

4
THE FANATIC

'A fool who thinks he is a fool is for that
very reason a wise man. The fool who thinks
he is wise is called a fool indeed.'

— Buddha, from the *Dhammapada*

Let's get one thing straight. Being fanatical is not always a bad thing. The Fanatic often sticks to a strict code or ethos and likes to feel in control. Who doesn't at least sometimes? The Fanatic needs something to hold on to, to belong to, an identity that makes them feel right. Being a fanatic only becomes a problem when we start to believe that there is no other way to live, and if we move a little to the left or right, failure will set in.

The Fanatic often bursts with unwavering enthusiasm and critical zeal. It's called . . . passion. Almost everyone has a belief or interest that gets them fired up, so really, we're all fanatics of some sort. It only gets dangerous when the principle encompasses The Fanatic's entire being, and becomes so all-important that he or she becomes rigid in their views. Natural medicine experts believe that rigidity in the mind causes acidity in our bodies, and we often see that fanaticism can actually conceal a hatred of some kind. If you see yourself as a little fanatical, ask yourself: are you poisoning yourself by being too rigid?

Consider this Japanese proverb: 'The bamboo that bends is stronger than the oak that resists.' The bamboo is flexible and adaptable, which allows it to bend and sway. But if you're rigid like an oak, you could snap at the first sign of resistance.

MENTAL FLEXIBILITY

1. Practise empathy: the ability to understand the emotional state of others and desire to alleviate the suffering of others. This involves getting out of a rut and doing something purely for the greater good.

2. Life begins at the end of your comfort zone. Try doing and seeing things a different way.

3. Beauty is in the soul, not in the face. Win friends with kindness and humility, not your ability to win an argument.

4. Don't take yourself too seriously – learn to relax and laugh more. You deserve to have some fun, too.

5. Allow yourself to make mistakes – mistakes are simply lessons in life. We have to make mistakes to learn and grow.

6. Examine your fears, which are only fears because that's how you perceive them. Only you can transform your perception so you no longer fear that object, outcome or feeling.

7. Practise random acts of kindness. Enrich the lives of others, if only in a small way. Your own life will become more enriched – guaranteed.

8. If you're fanatical about food, ask yourself, 'What's the worst thing that will happen to me if I have this slice of brie/glass of champagne/scoop of gelato?' Food should make you feel good, not guilty.

9. Know that 'purity' is not just about detoxifying your body, but your mind as well. Buddhists believe your body is an out-picturing of your thoughts. We must seek out negative thinking and fill it with positive, alkalising thoughts.

10. Party once in a while. Life is to be enjoyed, not endured, so put on your dancing shoes and party like there's no tomorrow!

CLEANSING DRINKS

LIVER CLEANSE

This drink is excellent for regenerating your liver as it helps flush out toxins. The Liver Flush Drink also assists in the release of metabolic acids, helps in the removal of excess fat and can help with the elimination of gallstones by normalising bile production. Blend all the ingredients on high for 15 seconds and drink immediately. It's best taken just before bed for three consecutive nights.

- 125 ml olive oil
- 125 ml orange, lemon or grapefruit juice
- 1 bulb garlic
- 4 cm piece fresh ginger root
- 2 pinches cayenne pepper

PARASITE CLEANSE

Parasites, worms and other pathogens can infest the digestive system and cause upsets, especially giardiasis, gastroenteritis and gastrointestinal candidiasis. The most potent parasite cleanses available need to be made up by a naturopath and should include herbs such as black walnut hull, horopito, wormwood, pau d'arco, citrus seed extract, fennel and goldenseal. Please note that parasitic cleanses should not be taken if you're pregnant or breastfeeding.

THE BREATH OF LIFE

Correct, deep breathing brings more oxygen to your cells and expels more carbon dioxide. Naturopaths also believe that it allows our bodies to regenerate by making our blood pH alkaline. It is really important to use your nose (not mouth) to inhale, as the tiny hairs in your nose helps filter the air before it reaches your lungs.

As you draw in each breath, expand your belly outwards, instead of raising your chest upwards. Imagine your trunk is an empty cavern or a balloon that's being filled with air. As you exhale, through the nose or the mouth, suck your belly in and deflate the proverbial balloon. This is called 'diaphragm breathing': it draws the diaphragm further down to give your lungs room to expand in every direction. When you breathe out, the diaphragm relaxes and air is effortlessly pushed out of your lungs. Diaphragm breathing goes hand-in-hand with posture, so if you really want to fill your lungs, sit up straight with your shoulders back. Ever seen a slouchy yogi? Didn't think so!

Mouth breathing over a long period of time will result in shorter and shallower breaths, which directly affects the amount of oxygen that can enter and therefore alkalise our blood. This in turn alters our posture as the brain interprets shallow breathing as breathing difficulty, and attempts to adjust by trying to open our airways.

Chest breathing has a similar effect on our posture as it forces the muscles of the chest and shoulders to contract, compensating for the lack of air that is able to enter our bodies. Furthermore, breathing from the chest only ever allows air to be delivered to the top part of our lungs, making us work harder to take in more breaths. Diaphragmatic breathing on the other hand, requires much less effort; when we breathe in from the diaphragm, it automatically contracts and enlarges our chest cavity. This enlargement creates a kind of suction, reducing the pressure inside and drawing air into the lungs. When we breathe out, the diaphragm relaxes and air is effortlessly pushed out.

You can't do this all the time, I know. When you're running for the bus or sprinting after a football, for example, you're likely to gulp for air through your mouth. And when your body's in fight or flight mode, you're naturally inclined to breathe with the chest.

Dr Andrew Weil, Ph. D, natural health practitioner, world-renowned speaker and author of many books on health says, 'If I had to limit my advice on healthier living to just one tip, it would be simply to learn how to breathe correctly.' And yogis say, 'Quality of breath, quality of mind.'

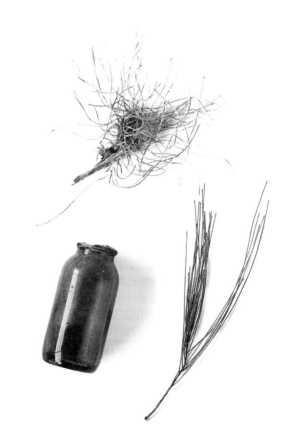

YOGA

Yoga means 'union', referring to the connection between mind and body through awareness of the breath. By aligning the breath with the practice of asanas (postures), you can become more aware of long-held tensions – physically and mentally. Through regular yoga practice, you can learn to let go of these tight spots, simply by breathing deeply and stretching the body. Natural medicine experts believe that yoga is deeply alkalising; it also provides us with tools for life. Learning to control the breath in awkward poses and watching what emotions come up for us helps us to deal with how we respond to the challenges of everyday life.

There are many forms of yoga. Studios are on every second street corner and new disciplines are emerging all the time. So it's important to choose a style that suits you – not because the DVD is on sale. Your yoga style will change as your needs change. If you're super-active and love your sport, look for a style that's more calming and reflective, such as Hatha, Iyengar, Satyananda or Yin. If you sit in front of a computer all day, you might enjoy a more dynamic and invigorating practice such as Asthanga, Bikram or Power yoga. Kundalini is a powerful discipline that aims to awaken dormant energy at the base of the spine. Other beautiful styles include Vinyasa, Jivamukti, Anusara and Shakti Dance, which focus on the graceful, dance-like aspects of yoga.

HEAVY METAL DETOX

Unfortunately, heavy metals are part of our lives, from fossil fuel combustion, car exhaust, batteries and wood burning, to the fish we eat and even the water we drink. Heavy metal overload may disrupt the endocrine system, which is in charge of hormone regulation and brain function. This, in turn, can lead to tumours and neurological problems. (There's a theory that milliners once used mercury to treat animal pelts, which made them schizophrenic – hence 'mad as a hatter'.)

When it comes to fish, you should limit the large, predatory varieties such as shark, ray, swordfish, orange roughy, gemfish, ling and barramundi, and big-eye, yellowfin and southern blue-fin tuna. Because they're at the top of the food chain, these species accumulate more mercury. I believe that bottom-feeders such as prawns, scallops, lobster and crab need to be limited as well.

Smaller species of tuna are used in the tinned variety, so you can safely snack on that twice a week. Salmon, snapper, sardines, whiting, garfish, mackerel and other cold-water oily fish are also considered low-mercury.

The following foods and supplements may help counteract heavy metal overload.

- Parsley and coriander: these humble herbs work as powerful chelation agents, helping to remove harmful toxins such as lead, aluminium and mercury from the brain.

- Vitamin C: a powerful antioxidant and immunity booster.

- DMSA (dimercaptosuccinic acid): especially good at mopping up mercury and lead. It works by binding with heavy metal molecules which are then excreted through the kidneys. DMSA needs to be administered by a health practitioner.

- Superoxide dismutase (or SOD): possibly the most potent antioxidant available. It's an enzyme that negates the effects of heavy metals by healing free radical damage.

- Amla (Embolic officinalis) – high in vitamin C, this counteracts the toxic effects of heavy metals when taken regularly.

PETE MELOV, *live food activist*

I've always loved the sun, being active, climbing trees and anything that involves being outside. I was pretty healthy as a kid, never drank coffee or tea, and was really not interested in sweets much. My downfall was white bread, and I smoked pot for a long time till about 20 years ago, when I gave it all up: sugar, refined foods, alcohol and drugs. I don't have a mobile phone and won't get one!

First thing every day, I get up and stretch. I take about 30 deep breaths in and out through my nose, as this activates numerous pathways through your sense of smell, and of course expels the toxins that might have built up in your lungs overnight. Next is a dry brush of my skin, and I brush my hair 100 times to stimulate my scalp. I like to massage with apple cider vinegar. I then practise the Tibetan Five Rites – awesome balancing exercises. I haven't missed a day since 1999! I then do a digestive cleanse called The Salt Purge, which cleans my digestive tract and colon. I love feeling clean; it gives me so much energy and balance.

I don't eat breakfast, I just do the purge. A lot of people mistake thirst for hunger – I find that when I am hydrated, I never feel hungry.

I usually fast until 1 or 2 p.m. every day and yes, I have loads of energy! I eat salads, raw organic eggs, some homemade bread. I always put a bit of nigari (aka magnesium chloride) in my water with some Celtic sea salt or Himalayan rock salt. I eat small amounts of raw lamb or chicken, and I love fermented foods.

My tips for optimum health are: eat chemical-free food and cleanse regularly. Fast periodically to remove all chemicals from your system. Talk to your neighbours and be part of your community. If possible, get rid of your radio, TV and newspapers, and start creating a positive mindset by knowing who you are. Slow down, eat slowly and chew your food to liquid before you swallow. Drink lots of good pH water as you never know if that hunger is really thirst. Remember, you are not that person with the big car and the big bank account. Look in the mirror: do you see yourself or just a reflection? Know that your inner world is important, not your exterior. Get outside as much as possible, treasure nature and the sun: we are meant to be sun-kissed. We *are* nature, so live as naturally as possible.

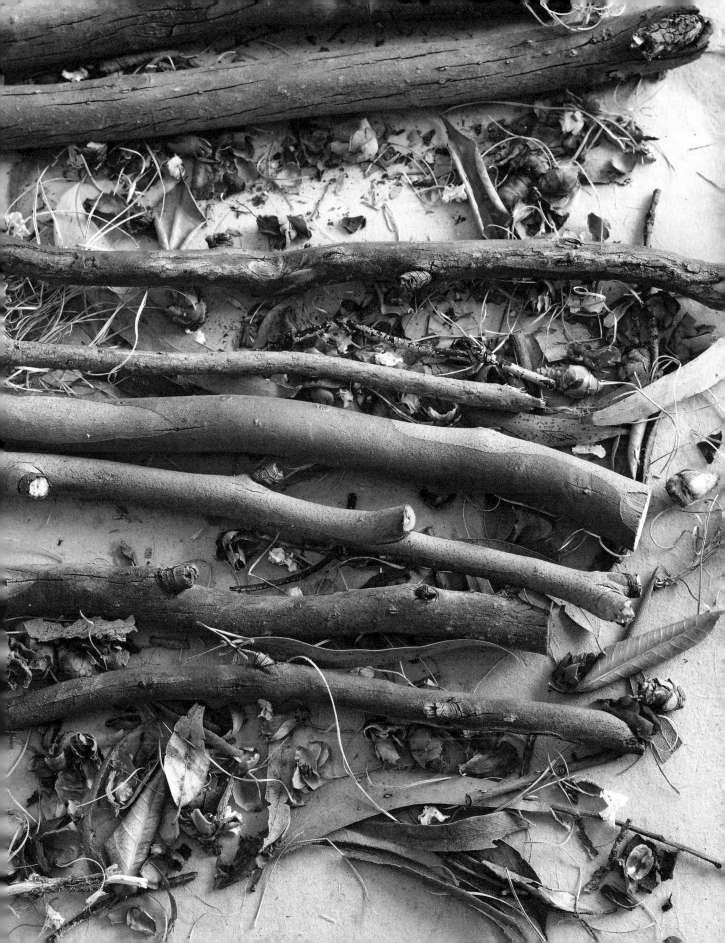

5
THE MAMAS & THE PAPAS

'Things that are truly of merit require time
and patience in order to be fulfilled.'
— Swami Kripalu

Doesn't your life change when you have kids? From your ability to function on zero sleep to your inherent values, things will never quite be the same after you bring children into the world. Your capacity for patience and appreciation of the smallest wonders in life grows, not to mention your relationship with your partner, family and yourself. You'll remember what it's like to jump in puddles or colonise a Lego city. Children make us happy, they make us angry, they definitely teach us about relentlessness and they are divine miracles.

To be a good parent and keep up with your kids, you must find time for yourself. You know the expression, 'Happy wife, happy life'? Well, 'Happy mum, happy baby' couldn't be more true (the same goes for dads, too). If you become a martyr and put yourself last, your children will suffer for it, simply because you're rattier with them and with your partner.

Once upon a time, in societies all around the world, children were brought up by the community. You know the saying, 'It takes a village to bring up a child.' We're still doing it, only now we pay for community care through childcare, babysitters and nannies. Our mental and emotional wellbeing is partly dependent on an authentic sense of community. Get to know and love your neighbour's children; ask the elderly lady from across the road if she needs any groceries; host a block party. If you learn to help others, then when you need assistance, you'll be in a better position to ask for it.

Children are our teachers, not the other way around. In the extraordinarily beautiful and wise words of Kahlil Gibran in *The Prophet*, 'Your children are not your children. They are sons and daughters of Life's longing for itself. They come through you but not from you, and though they are with you, yet they belong not to you.' Amen.

CREATING HEALTHY KIDS

1   Children pay attention not to what you say, but what you do. They will eat and drink what you eat and drink. If you don't want them to eat something, don't eat it yourself.

2   Whether you like it or not, kids are little reflections of us. If they're grumpy, look in the mirror. Are *you* grumpy? If they're competitive, is it because you are?

3   Eat wholefoods 85 per cent of the time: the less processed the food, the easier it is on your child's digestive system. Natural medicine experts believe that the genetically modified ingredients, additives and preservatives found in processed foods are among the main causes of the increase of allergies and intolerances prevalent today.

4   Behavioural problems have been linked with the preservative calcium propionate (282), commonly used in bread. Always check labels for long lists of numbers and unpronounceable ingredients, as childhood diseases such as asthma, hyperactivity and learning difficulties are often linked with these food additives.

5   Don't be too strict with children; otherwise you'll have a serious rebellion on your hands when they're teenagers.

6   Children love and thrive on routine. Eating, playing, napping and going to bed at a similar time every day will make for happier and more contented kids.

7   Ensure your baby's bottle and kids' drink bottles are BPA-free: a Harvard study suggests that exposure to plastics made with the chemical bisphenol A (BPA) can disrupt the endocrine system.

8   Spend quality time with your kids. Turn off computers, phones and iPads and play. Before you know it, they'll be grown up and won't want to hang out with you!

9   It's your responsibility to get your child out and about, rather than sitting indoors playing with gadgets.

10 Take time out for yourself without feeling guilty – children are more resilient than you think and you'll be a better parent for it.

KITCHEN HEALERS

Sure, herbs in tincture form (dispensed by your naturopath or herbalist) are the most potent, but you can use everyday herbs from your pantry or kitchen garden to give your family a healthy boost.

Basil: is great for concentration and lifting your mood. Also has antibacterial and anti-inflammatory properties.

Cacao: theobromine, found in chocolate, translates as 'food of the gods'. It's filled with antioxidants and has mood-lifting qualities; darker varieties of raw cacao are best.

Chamomile: it's antibacterial, soothes tummy aches and calms whingey children.

Chilli and cayenne pepper: warming herbs that are great for weight loss. Chilli in particular is known also as a febrifuge, which heats up the body for a speedy recovery from fever.

Cinnamon: antiseptic and soothing to the digestive system. Maintains blood sugar levels and eases nausea and vomiting.

- Cloves: a great parasite cleanser. Placing a clove bud on an aching tooth will ease the pain; also works as an antiseptic.

- Fennel: eat fennel seeds with a pinch of sea salt for indigestion, flatulence, nausea, morning sickness and cystitis.

- Fenugreek: soak seeds overnight in water and drink the infused water the next morning to ease symptoms of excessive gas and bloating.

- Garlic: nature's antibiotic; great for the common cold and tummy upsets. For earaches, crush raw garlic, mix with olive or mullein oil and strain. Then drop the liquid into the ear. Block it with cotton wool and leave overnight.

- Ginger: boasts anti-inflammatory qualities and improves circulation. Widely used for motion and morning sickness, nausea and indigestion.

- Lavender: used for everything from anxiety, insomnia and depression to indigestion and colic. Also works well as a mosquito repellent.

- Liquorice root: great for coughs and bronchitis. Also a good option to ease symptoms of constipation and stress.

- Oregano: great for coughs and colds. Also an anti-fungal and can be used topically for skin conditions such as psoriasis.

- Parsley and coriander: boast the ability to remove heavy metals from your body.

- Peppermint: alleviates tummy aches, indigestion and colic.

- Rosemary: a wonderful antioxidant and antidepressant. Also used for poor concentration and memory.

- Sage: an antiseptic for the mouth and throat; makes a wonderful gargle for tonsillitis and gingivitis.

- Thyme: an antibacterial and anthelmintic (it kills worms). Try Kick-a-Germ juice (recipe on p 144) for colds and flus. Also used for asthma and bronchitis.

- Turmeric: a potent antioxidant with anti-inflammatory qualities. Curcumin, the active ingredient in turmeric, is used in the treatment of cancer.

FOOD LABELS

Most packaged foods have a label listing their ingredients and nutritional content: energy (kilojoules or calories); carbohydrates; sugar; salt or sodium; fats; fibre and protein. The ingredients list is in descending order: the ingredient with the largest amount goes first, while the ingredient with the smallest amount is last. For example, if sugar is second on the list of muesli bar ingredients, ahead of nuts, fruit and whole wheat, put it back on the supermarket shelf.

You've probably seen many brands make nutritional claims, such as '99 per cent fat-free!' 'No added sugar!', 'High in fibre!' or 'Low in cholesterol!'. Be careful with these products. Fat-free could really mean 'Full of sugar!' and no added sugar doesn't mean the food is low in kilojoules. Seemingly healthy packaged foods might also contain artificial sweeteners or transfats.

Preservatives do exactly that: they're chemicals that extend the shelf life of a packaged food. Food colouring is used to make stuff look more palatable and other additives enhance taste (isn't food tasty enough?). Also referred to as 'excitotoxins', some additives have been implicated in behavioural and health problems, and allergies, in kids. For a comprehensive list of excitotoxins, chemicals and food additives, I recommend Bill Statham's book *The Chemical Maze* (Possibility.com).

KEEP THEM ACTIVE

Depression and mental health issues are growing concerns in today's society. According to Australian research, children are 35 per cent less likely to suffer from depression in adulthood if they're physically active. Why? Exercise stimulates the brain to produce more neurotransmitters such as serotonin and endorphins, or 'happy hormones'. Since little ones' brains develop so much in childhood, the effect could be greater than in grown-ups. Movement also boosts brain proteins while reducing oxidative stress. But wait, there's more! Sport in particular teaches kids important social and cognitive skills from an early age, such as teamwork, learning to share, and hand-eye coordination.

BUY ORGANIC

1   Children's health: little ones are more susceptible to the nasties from pesticide residues and environmental toxins as their organs are still developing.

2   Optimal nutrition: because organic farmers use less water, crops are seasonal with fewer early pickings. Reduced storage time means fruit and veg is more nutrient-rich.

3   Animal welfare: organic farming is ethical, meaning animals are free to roam and not treated with antibiotics or hormones. Cattle are fed grass, which is better suited to their digestive system than (non-organic) grains.

4   Environmental protection: sustainable agriculture uses fewer fossil fuels, thereby producing fewer carbon dioxide emissions. Organic farming protects our soil and water, ensuring a safer planet for our kids.

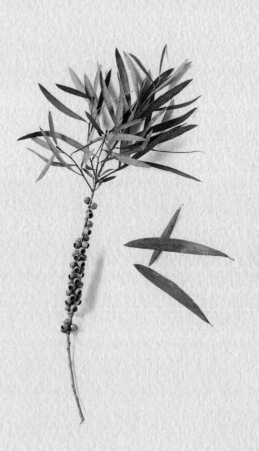

CAMILLA FREEMAN-TOPPER,

fashion designer, Camilla and Marc

I have always tried to lead a fairly balanced lifestyle. I have had the business since I was twenty-one, so I've always had big responsibilities on a day-to-day basis. This has probably helped me to keep things balanced.

I try to eat reasonably well; however, I do love savoury food. Both my kids and I love eggs, so a few days a week I cook up a big breakfast for us with eggs, spinach and mushrooms or capsicum. On the other days I tend to eat porridge in winter and cereal in summer. Because I eat early in the morning with them, I tend to eat lunch early as well. I try to mix it up so either salads, sushi or pasta. I love to cook in the evenings so I'll make steak or veal scaloppini, roasted or steamed vegies, fish, pasta or a big salad for dinner. I don't like to eat huge dinners because my breakfasts are usually so big. I don't drink coffee so I drink lots of water with lemon or green teas and at least one fresh juice a day.

I have recently found a new love in jogging while pushing my baby in the pram. I tend to mix up walking and running in the same routine and I usually try to get out at least three days a week. Before the girls were born, I used to do lots of yoga and Pilates, but because I have so little time I find it harder to get to a class these days. I hope to return to Pilates in summer, but in the meantime, jogging and walking will absolutely suffice.

Australians are lucky to have the incredible landscape we live in. On any day of the year, even in winter, it's never too cold to get out and go for a walk or jog at the beach.

Good health is a true gift, so everything you can do to stay healthy is very important. Saying that, I am not someone to obsess about being super-fit; I really believe it's about a good balance. So having a glass or two of wine to unwind, or eating something that isn't necessarily the healthiest is good to do once in a while.

When I feel a flu coming on, eating good, nutritious food always helps to kick it quickly. Plus drinking lots of water, eating fresh fruit and vegetables and maintaining a balanced lifestyle.

I'm a huge believer in children eating a healthy, balanced diet and getting outdoors as often as possible. It's so important for their little bodies to be fed well with very little junk food and go to the park for a run around to exert their energy. One thing I learnt very early on when my first child was a baby was to ensure I was happy and healthy. I realised that if I didn't make time to eat good food or do exercise regularly, I wouldn't be the mother I wanted to be. We are so time-poor these days, so the more organised you can be to make time for yourself, the better mother you are for your children.

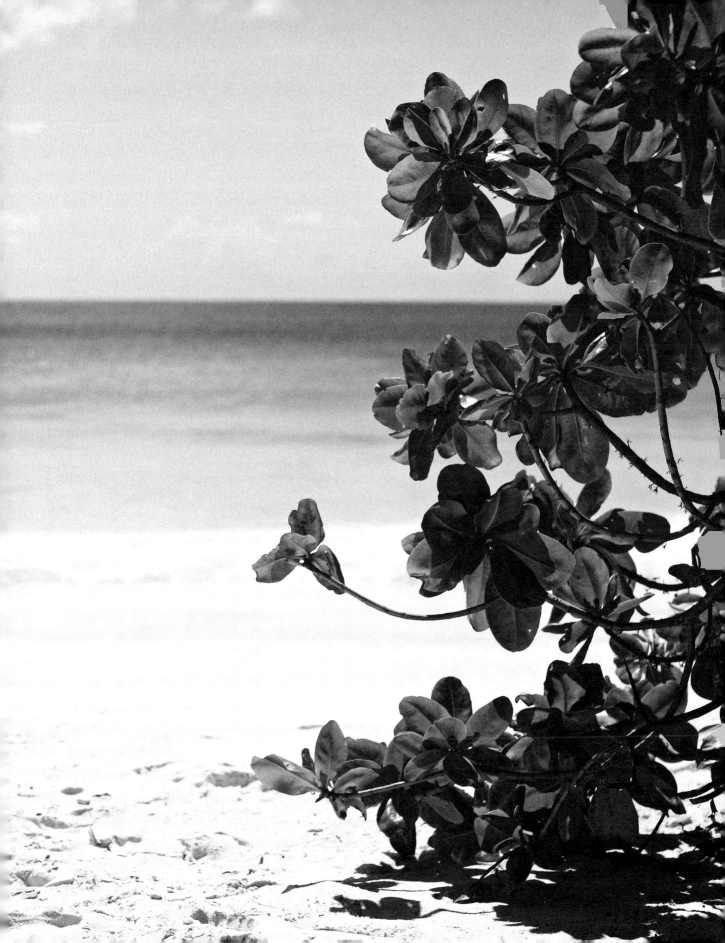

6
THE YOUNG AT HEART

'It is never too late to be
what you might have been.'

— George Eliot

Everyone seems to be worried sick about ageing. The explosion of anti-ageing supplements, beauty products and treatments (including invasive cosmetic treatments) form a growing multi-billion-dollar industry. But ageing is part and parcel of life, and the wonderful thing about growing older is self-acceptance and wisdom. You no longer sweat the small stuff. You can let go of regret and ego-driven behaviour. Hopefully, as you age you naturally become more in touch with your soul.

In your golden years, you might have more time for your family, friends and yourself. If you choose to wind down work, your schedule can be liberated. It's the time when you can really enjoy the fruits of your labour. You might find time to help within the community, do volunteer work or discover a new passion.

Age is most definitely a state of mind. If you see yourself as old, you will feel and look old. But you can empower yourself by seeing ageing as a natural progression. No matter how many facelifts you get or sports cars you buy, you can't actually stop the clock. Accept this fact and growing old will not seem like a disease that you have to treat, but a time of spiritual gifts such as wisdom and compassion.

As we age, our bodily functions naturally slow down and the ability to eliminate toxins and acids may reduce. I believe the accumulation of these waste products is the main cause of the visible signs of ageing. Because the harmful by-products cannot be efficiently released, the body stores them in organs and fat, giving rise to a host of conditions such as high cholesterol, heart disease, arthritis and osteoporosis.

I can't say it enough: eat alkalising food, hydrate properly and detoxify regularly – body and mind – to cut this free radical damage. You'll increase your body's capability to dispose of wastes. This is the only sure-fire way to slow down the signs of ageing; what's more, it's completely free!

AGEING WELL

1 Follow a diet of alkalising, whole and unprocessed foods.

2 Go for 50 per cent raw food. As digestion slows down in later years, the body's ability to produce digestive enzymes is impaired; naturopaths believe raw foods provide the body with much-needed enzymes to break down food.

3 Cut back on sugar: sugars increase free radicals called AGES (advanced glycation end products), which accelerate ageing on the inside and out.

4 Focus on fibre: a high-fibre diet is important as we age due to a slowing of the digestive system.

5 Detox regularly: give your liver a holiday. Like any organ, the liver ages and becomes more sluggish at processing toxins as time goes on.

6 Move your body: it's the quickest route to mental and emotional wellbeing, and will help prevent osteoporosis and injuries.

7 Mind stimulation activities: keep your brain's synapses firing and stave off Alzheimer's disease and dementia.

8 Be kind to yourself: remember that ageing is a natural process; staying youthful and beautiful is an attitude.

9 Don't go plastic: it's obvious and looks terrible. Age gracefully!

10 Socialise: join a club, take up a hobby, volunteer. Now you've got more time, use it.

FIBRE FACTS

Just as you drink water, exercise and brush your teeth, make eating fibre a part of your daily routine. Not only does fibre help with digestion and elimination, it can lower cholesterol, promote beneficial gut flora and make you feel fuller for longer. To increase your fibre:

- Eat raw vegetables in the form of salads, crudités and sprouts.

- Eat nuts, seeds, whole grains and sprouted breads. Oatmeal, bran and barley are also great sources of fibre.

- Add peas, beans and lentils to soups, casseroles and salads.

- Eat whole fruits instead of drinking juice.

- Add one tablespoon of chia seeds, flaxseed or LSA meal to your Go Green Juice (see recipe on p 142).

- Reduce your consumption of meat, sweets and processed foods to 15 per cent of your food intake, as these are low in fibre.

- For extra fibre, try 1–2 teaspoons of psyllium husks in warm water at night before bed.

USE YOUR BRAIN

- Crosswords, sudoku puzzles and jigsaws may help strengthen brain cells by lengthening connective fibres in the brain.

- Take up a hobby – gardening, learning to play a musical instrument, playing poker – it doesn't really matter. Discovering new skills enhances cognitive function and increases memory.

Read more (and watch less TV). Reading stimulates the imagination whereas television does not.

Take up dancing – not only is it fun and social, it's a perfect way to stitch up the mind-body connection.

Sleep more. Sleep is restorative, it increases your ability to learn and keeps your hormones in check.

STAY ACTIVE

Unfortunately, with age comes a susceptibility to injuries because of the natural loss of strength, balance and flexibility. Of course, we can increase our chances if we move our bodies regularly throughout our lives. You don't need to be a record-breaking ageing marathoner or, at the other end of the spectrum, to don the whites and take up lawn bowls. Just staying active will improve circulation, ward off heart disease, protect your mental health (endorphins!) and keep you looking and feeling younger. Here are my suggestions:

Low-impact yoga is fantastic for maintaining strength and flexibility; it helps improve balance, which will prevent falls. Yogis say that you can tell the age of a person by the flexibility of their spine.

Pilates works the core muscles, so it helps correct posture and protects against injury.

Swimming works all the muscle groups, increases cardiovascular fitness and is easy on the joints.

Walking at a moderate pace for 45 minutes (or more) each day boosts cardiovascular health, builds strength and takes you outdoors.

Tai chi enhances the mind-body connection, balance, flexibility and strength by igniting the 'chi' (energy) in your body.

ANTI-AGEING SUPPLEMENTS

Astragalus (*Astragalus membranaceus*): used frequently in Chinese medicine to combat signs of ageing. An immunity-boosting herb that can help prevent colds and respiratory infections, as well as lowering blood pressure.

DHEA (*dehydroepiandrosterone*) & HGH (*Human Growth Hormone*) – DHEA and HGH levels decline as we age, however, there are risks associated with taking HGH injections. DHEA, on the other hand, is an intermediate substance which is converted into HGH by the adrenal glands, therefore the body only makes as much HGH as it requires, without causing disturbances to the other systems in the body.

Fulvic acid: touted as 'the miracle molecule' because of its ability to regenerate all cells in the body. It is the element that help you absorb nutrients.

Gotu kola (*Centella asiatica*): Indians say, 'Two leaves of gotu kola a day keeps ageing at bay.'

Methyl Sulfonyl Methane (MSM): a sulphur-containing compound which helps to build and maintain healthy connective tissues, useful for arthritis and muscle pain. Food sources include eggs, broccoli, beans, lean beef, poultry, soybeans, cabbage, clams, fish, milk, kale, brussels sprouts, garlic, onions, and whole wheat.

- Mushroom extract: has long been used in traditional Chinese medicine for everything from recovery from chronic illnesses to upper respiratory tract infections and recurrent candidiasis.

- Resveratrol (*Polygonum cuspidatum*): boasts antioxidant and anti-inflammatory properties. It's also found naturally in grape skins and dark chocolate.

- SAMe and TMG: S-adenosylmethionine and trimethylglycine both improve liver function and may alleviate depression. TMG is the less expensive form and helps the body create its own SAMe.

- Selenium: a powerful antioxidant, also known for its anti-cancer qualities. Food sources include seafood, including kelp and seaweed, onion, garlic, broccoli, tuna, eggs and brazil nuts. Do not exceed 600mcg daily.

- Silica: my favourite brand is Orgono Living Silica, a silica supplement which increases the mobility and functioning of joints and cartilage. Also increases collagen production and skin elasticity.

| CASE STUDY |

CHRISTINE MANFIELD,

chef, author and restaurateur

Staying healthy means keeping in tune with my body and responding to its needs. Being aware of how my body works and how I can keep it working at its optimum; not succumbing to weakness. I make sure I take regular exercise (a mix of cardio, weight-training and yoga), stay young at heart, engage with the world and what's going on around me, and have a positive attitude. I have introduced Saimaa's detox and cleansing diet into my way of life and do it regularly to get my body functioning more efficiently, to combat age and feel the best I possibly can. Regular visits to my chiropractor and acupuncturist keep everything in check.

When it comes to ageing, I say: don't act your age! A good dose of silliness goes a long way. Make sure you have fun – every day. Don't use cosmetic surgery to interfere with nature's progress – natural beauty gives you that inner glow. Don't obsess about ageing. It's inevitable, but at the same time there are a few easy things you can do to feel and look younger. Protecting your skin is key: using moisturiser is an everyday ritual for me; I use factor 30+ sunblock when I'm in the sun, and I get my skin checked regularly by a dermatologist.

The secret to ageing gracefully, as far as I'm concerned, is eating well, preparing fresh food, eschewing fast foods and instant, highly processed foods in favour of organic, sustainable and natural produce. Get regular, strenuous exercise to keep physically fit, mentally alert and engaged. Seek out challenges and laugh a lot. Humour is healthy.

'The foolish are careless and negligent
but the wise carry out every detail
with mindfulness.'

— Buddha

Despite the name, Enlightened Beings don't take themselves too seriously. They have a relaxed approach to health and probably already live by the principles and secrets of the Aussie Body Diet. They know that true health is not just about putting nutritious food and drink into their bodies; it has to encompass the mind and spirit, as well as the body.

Sound like you? If you're an Enlightened Being, I'm guessing you already commit to regular detoxes. You know this is important for optimal, permanent health. You know that taking time out for yourself is vital for a clear head and a clean body. You're aware that reflective contemplation time allows you to be in touch with your spirit. I'm preaching to the converted!

Let's just rehash some of the finer details: the philosophies that can enrich the lives of anyone – The Hedonist, The Athlete, The Young at Heart – all of us. Always remember that negative thoughts and emotions are natural – they arise in all of us – but try not to allow negativity to shake the goodness in you. Thoughts come and go. Make the conscious decision not to attach yourself to the negative feelings. Enlightened Beings don't judge, even when people judge them. Judgement, criticising and idle gossip are a reflection of insecurity. It's a negative, toxic habit. So some people use anger as a weapon. So what? You don't have to.

Make a habit of tuning into your own internal commentary; convert negative thoughts into positive, constructive affirmations. Practise mindfulness: real power is not power over others, but power over one's self. Strive to be happy. If you've come from a horrendous childhood or survived an abusive relationship, anger and bitterness won't take you far. Forgiveness, on the other hand, will set you free. Keep honing that mind control; attract only what you want in your life. It will come to you, as long as you keep stepping with grace and poise. Harness gratitude, humility and compassion. Remember, true radiant beauty is a lightness of being. Yes, you look good because you eat well, work out and detox. But that glow every cosmetics company in the world wants to bottle? It comes from balancing the mind, body and spirit.

MINIMISE TOXINS

1   Grooming products: your skin is a protective barrier and one of our vital elimination channels. It matters, so always choose a toxin-free brand or make your own using natural emollients and essential oils.

2   Household cleaning products: seek out safe cleaning solutions, such as eucalyptus oil, tea tree oil, bicarbonate of soda and white vinegar.

3   Oxygenate your home: surround yourself with indoor plants and open the windows when you can to ensure your home gets fresh air.

4   Purchase a water ioniser. It's an outlay at first but only requires non-costly maintenance once a year.

5   Switch your mobiles, smart phones, cordless phones and computers off regularly to avoid radiation exposure. Check out the latest anti-radiation technology from companies like Aulterra.

6   Cook only in stainless-steel, cast-iron, glass or high-quality enamel cookware to reduce heavy metal exposure.

7   Clothe your family in organic fibres, which further reduce your contact with toxins. They're also better for the environment.

8   Use whole grains and nuts that have been prepared by soaking, sprouting or fermenting to neutralise phytic acid and help repopulate good bacteria in the gut.

9   Commit to the Aussie Body 14-day Diet twice a year. It's not purely for your physical self, but also your mental, emotional and spiritual selves.

10 After the program, continue to practise the habits you learned in the Maintenance Phase.

MIND AND SPIRIT REMEDIES

•   Brahmi (*Bacopa monneiri*) is an Ayurvedic herb used for its mind-boosting properties. Traditionally the Brahmis used this herb to promote mental alertness while inducing a sense of calm and peace.

•   Ormus has been reported to cure serious diseases such as multiple sclerosis, arthritis and even cancer. It may increase your spiritual connection, heighten intuition and perception, and boost overall consciousness.

•   Tulsi (*Ocinum santum*): also known as 'holy basil', this is one of the most sacred plants in India. It is believed to have blood-purifying qualities, and it also strengthens immunity, calms the mind and improves mental ability.

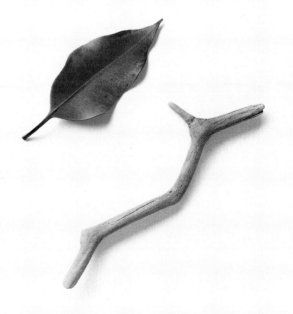

ON INTUITION

It is said that your intuition is your spirit talking to you, guaranteeing you the right perspective if you choose to listen. Some of us hear the spirit but the mind quickly takes over, colouring intuition with rational thought. Ever ignored your intuition and later on said, 'I knew it!' or 'I knew I should have . . .'

Harnessing the power of intuition comes from having a sense of both your heart and your head. Pay more attention to what your heart tells you and practise clearing your mind. Ask for guidance. Trust that it will point you in the right direction.

MEDITATION

Meditation relaxes the body, increases your capacity to handle stressful situations and regenerates cells. Meditation improves physical, emotional and mental health. It gives you a sense of calm, clarity and concentration. Meditation does everything but rub your feet.

To meditate, set aside a time of the day when you know nothing is going to disturb you. Switch off the phone. Start with five or 10 minutes a day, working your way up to a longer session as it suits you. Or keep it short, if that's more sustainable.

- Sit comfortably on the ground, on a cushion or on a chair. If it feels right, sit cross-legged or in the lotus position (cross-legged but with your feet resting on your thighs). Make sure your spine is straight, but not tense.

- Rest your hands on your lap or in a 'mudra' (hand position – a nice easy one is to have your thumb meeting your pointer or middle finger).

- Close your eyes.

- Bring your focus to your breath and practise deep breathing from the diaphragm. If it helps to count, do so. Count up to a number between three and 10 on every inhalation and exhalation, stopping just briefly between in- and out-breaths.

- Alternatively, take a mental tour of your body, tensing and relaxing each part in turn.

- Some people find it helpful to repeat a mantra – a short, positive affirmation or word, or a sound such as 'ohm'.

- If you find your thoughts wandering, don't get annoyed with yourself. Simply watch the thoughts with no attachment and let them go. Bring your attention back to your breath and/or mantra.

- That's all there is to it. Regular meditation allows you to quieten your mind and before you know it, you'll be meditating for 30 minutes and it will feel as if no time has passed.

EAT SEASONALLY

Eating produce in season is how our hunter-gatherer ancestors survived. Technology has made it possible for us to eat strawberries and mangoes all year round, but there are many reasons why we should go back to only eating produce when it is in season. One is that seasonal fruit and veg are nutritionally abundant: their nutrients decrease considerably the longer they are left after picking. Another is that produce grown out of season is often sprayed with all sorts of nasties to make them look appetising. Once you feel and taste the difference – the flavour, ripeness, quality and value – you'll never go back to what has become the conventional way (which is actually pretty unconventional, if you ask me).

MAEVE DERMODY, *actress*

I was raised primarily as a vegetarian, with a lot of respect given to preparing and eating food. When I was 13 I got my first job in a health food shop, where I learnt about food as medicine and just listening to what is going on in my body. The other side of this is knowing when to indulge. And I do; I'm not rigid. I drink alcohol and eat chocolate, just not excessively.

My daily routine varies as much as my work does. When shooting a film the hours tend to be longer and more unpredictable. In the theatre I know the hours I have to work, and how much energy that demands, so I organise things accordingly. I try not to wake late. I'm also a student, so if I know I have the morning free I'll try and study. If I have lines to learn I'll do that. I love the late afternoon, especially dusk, so I try to go for a long walk or run near where I live or by the sea. That is heaven. As an actor, structure needs to sit inside supreme flexibility because things are always being rearranged.

I'm a big tea drinker, and a hot cup in the morning eases me into the day. In winter I seek warming foods like porridge with stewed fruit and nuts. In summer, muesli, yoghurt (biodynamic and local because I need to know the cows are being treated well) and fruit is great. I like flaxseed oil on cereal too. I drink a lot of water – probably 2–3 litres a day. I like to make fresh vegetable juice too, and coconut water smoothies.

Lunch is soup or salad – I like to use fresh, seasonal vegies, and I try to include a good source of vegetarian protein such as nuts, miso, tofu or tahini. Dinner depends on whether I'm cooking at home or eating out. On the whole though I'll have some sort of curry or stir-fry, or salad with either quinoa or brown rice. But a general inclination is green, green, green!

I've had a strong, regular yoga practice for the past eight years, and I take my mat everywhere. I love a long run when I'm in the mood, and I ride my bike or walk everywhere I can. Being on foot and discovering things is wonderful. It clears my head and inspires me.

To relax, I love hot baths, tea and film watching or reading. Also just hanging out with friends. A change of scenery always rewires my brain in the best possible way. My mum and her partner have a beautiful property on the south coast of NSW and I try and escape there as much as possible.

We live in one of the luckiest countries in the world, and it is a blessing to be able to focus on our health beyond just staying alive. Good health also increases the quality of our relationships. I feel that as long as you don't become obsessive, then being thoughtful about your own health, the health of others, and the health of the planet is important and life-sustaining.

To stay healthy, my top tip is to get out of your head and listen to your body and the way it changes. Our bodies need such different things at different times, and only we can know that. It takes an open, relaxed attitude to be receptive.

In Australia, we are surrounded by such diverse and stunning nature. To be outside swimming in the ocean or walking through the bush reminds us of how to be in nature. It expands us, and teaches us about our bodies.

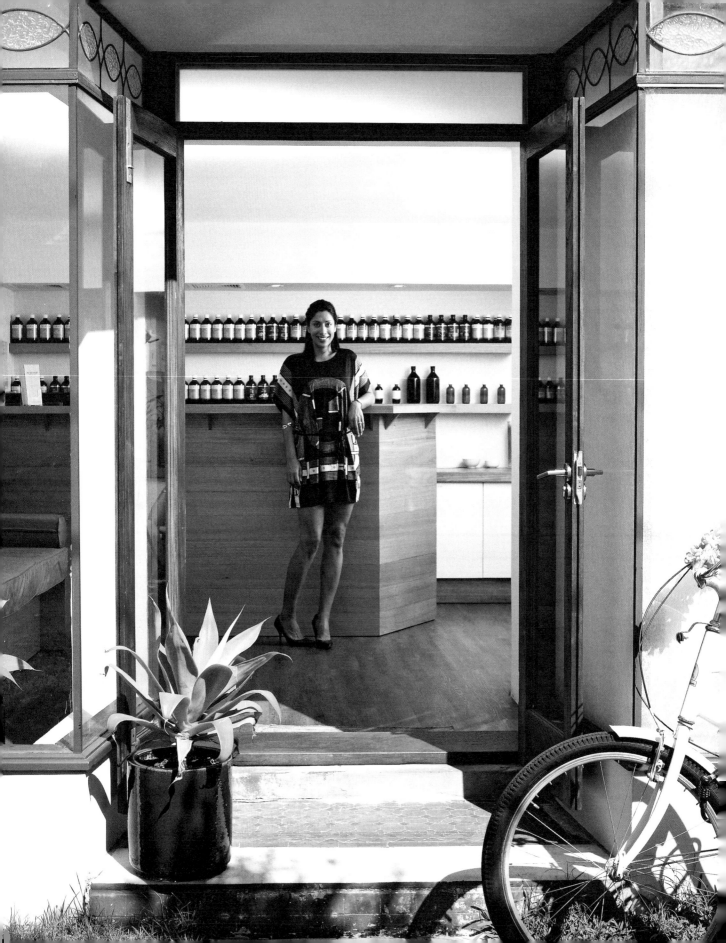

CONCLUSION

This book is a compendium of Australian lifestyle secrets. We have moved away from diets, counting calories, portion control, only eating protein or the low-carb fad. It is about looking good, feeling great and living a longer, more abundant life. It is about realising your true potential and understanding that optimum health and wellbeing has to encompass your physical, mental, emotional and spiritual states.

In my practice as a naturopath, I try to take into account the fact that life is cyclical, ever-changing and ever-transforming. Everything has its opposite: think of the sun and moon, day and night, love and hate, yin and yang. Each allows us to appreciate the other. This is why I have given you lifestyle secrets for different stages in your life, so you can address all your health, fitness and lifestyle needs, wherever you happen to be. This book exists to provide you with the real secrets for true health, optimum wellbeing, ultimate fitness and radiant beauty.

When you are healthy your eyes are bright, your skin is clear and glowing even without make-up, and your hair is naturally lustrous. When you are healthy, you'll be at your optimal body weight without having to starve yourself or restrict your diet. And most importantly, when you are healthy you treat yourself with love and respect, and therefore feel your best. The secret is when you 'feel' your best, that's when you look your hottest because you are radiating happiness and confidence, which is incredibly attractive.

To have a real Aussie Body and look and feel your absolute best, you must be healthy – remember, nothing feels as good as being healthy does.

It is well known globally that people in Australia take good care of our environment and of ourselves. It's because we have a great lifestyle, have instilled great habits and are eating to live!

This book is for everyone – children and adults, vegetarians, vegans, meat eaters and raw foodies. We have amazing secrets here in Australia and it's time we shared them with the world.

GUIDES & TOOLS

AUSSIE BODY 14-DAY PROGRAM CHECKLIST

DAILY	SUN	MON	TUE	WED	THU	FRI	SAT
Skin brushing							
Meditation/Breathing							
ACV/Cayenne shot							
Green drink							
7 SECRETS CHECKLIST							
Food							
Water							
Detox							
Movement							
Positive Outloook							
Sunlight							
Nature							
OPTIONAL							
Supplements							
Therapies							

See aussiebodydiet.com to print out more copies of the tables in this section.

DETOXIFICATION THERAPIES

Therapies are not only wonderful to indulge in, they also assist with detoxification processes by opening up elimination channels, improving circulation, de-stressing the body and assisting with lymph flow. Look for centres run by naturopaths as they tend to have a more holistic approach to therapies. Only use organic or natural products on your skin because it breathes and absorbs everything.

SKIN BRUSHING

Dry brushing exfoliates the skin, assists lymphatic drainage, strengthens the immune system and helps to tighten and tone skin. Skin brushing should be performed once a day, preferably first thing in the morning before showering. And make sure to clean your brush once a week using soap and water, then dry it in sunshine.

- Using a hard, natural fibre brush, begin with your feet and brush vigorously in circular motions up your legs.

- Proceed to your hands and arms.

- Brush your entire back (in an upwards direction) and abdomen area (using circular, counter-clockwise strokes), shoulders and neck (in a downwards direction).

- For women, lightly brush the breasts.

THERAPEUTIC MASSAGE

Massage allows you to release tension, assists circulation and supports the natural release of toxins. Regular massage strengthens and tones the entire body system. Deep-tissue, remedial and lymphatic massages should be part of a detox, as often as you like. For increased benefits, use organic coconut or sesame oil. I recommend regular massages on an ongoing basis, at least once a week.

COLON THERAPY

This ancient method of healing gently hydrates the colon and I believe it's the most effective treatment possible to detoxify the body, improve digestive function, clear out build-up and improve overall health.

Choose a reputable centre using the 'closed' system and only receive treatments from naturopaths, nutritionists or certified colon therapists – this will allow for optimum safety while cleansing and will guarantee an effective detoxification.

SALT THERAPY

Salt scrubs are not only divine to receive, they also improve skin texture, increase circulation and promote lymph flow. Some say they also cleanse the aura. Indulging in a salt scrub once a week is ideal during the program; choose only Epsom salt, coarse sea salt, Dead Sea mineral salt or Himalayan pink salt with emollients such as almond, sesame, coconut, olive or avocado oil, or cacao butter.

Salt scrubs are easy to do at home. Use four cups of one the salts listed above with one cup of one of the emollients listed above, and voila – you've made your own scrub, ready for a full body exfoliation. Shower afterwards, but soap is not necessary.

DETOX BODY WRAPS

Body wraps using mud, bentonite clay or seaweed detox the skin and help rid the body of excess fluids. A body wrap once a week is hugely beneficial during the program, and a motivating treat. You can try it at home: apply bentonite clay to your entire body, leave it on for at least twenty minutes and allow to harden. Then remove with a warm flannel, or better yet, with your DIY salt scrub!

ACID-ALKALINE CHART

FOOD CATEGORY	LEAST ALKALINE	ALKALINE	MOST ALKALINE	LEAST ACID	ACID	MOST ACID
Sweeteners	Raw honey, raw sugar	Maple syrup, rice syrup	Stevia	Processed honey, molasses	White sugar, brown sugar	Artificial sweeteners
Fruits	Oranges, bananas, cherries, pineapple, peaches, avocados	Dates, figs, melons, grapes, papaya, kiwi, blueberries, apples, pears, raisins	Lemons, watermelon, limes, grapefruit, mangoes, papayas	Plums, processed fruit juices	Sour cherries, rhubarb	Blackberries, cranberries, prunes
Nuts/Seeds	Chestnuts	Almonds		Pumpkin seeds, sunflower seeds	Pecans, cashews	Peanuts, walnuts
Beans Vegetables Legumes	Carrots, tomatoes, fresh corn, mushrooms, cabbage, peas, potato skins, olives, soybeans, tofu	Okra, squash, green beans, beets, celery, lettuce, zucchini, sweet potato, carob	Asparagus, onions, vegetable juices, watercress, parsley, raw spinach, broccoli, garlic	Cooked spinach, kidney beans, string beans	Potatoes (without skins), pinto beans, navy beans, lima beans	Chocolate
Oils	Canola oil	Flaxseed oil, Udo's 3-6-9 oil blend	Olive oil	Corn oil		
Grains Cereals	Amaranth, millet, wild rice, quinoa			Sprouted wheat bread, spelt, brown rice	White rice, corn, buckwheat, oats, rye	Wheat, white flour, pastries, pasta
Meats				Venison, cold water fish	Turkey, chicken, lamb	Beef, pork, shellfish
Eggs/Dairy	Soy cheese, soy milk, goat milk, goat cheese, whey	Breast milk		Eggs, butter, yoghurt, buttermilk, cottage cheese	Raw milk	Cheese, homogenised milk, ice cream
Beverages	Ginger tea	Green tea	Herb teas, lemon water	Tea	Coffee	Wine, beer, spirits, soft drinks
Habits	Optimism, rest, naps, fun, play, yoga and activities that relax you, clearing the mind, sleep, fresh air, loving and being loved, contentment, happiness, exercise, laughter, joyful emotions, expressions of joy, breathing deeply.			Anger, rage, complaining, nagging, envy, obsessive jealousy, fear and anxiety, gossip and backbiting, hateful emotions, dreams of revenge, shallow breathing, holding your breath, going without sleep, lack of exercise, overwork, pessimism.		

PROTEIN

GENERAL PROTEIN ESTIMATIONS

Most people need 0.8–1.0 g of protein per kilogram of body weight per day.			
100 g chicken breast (with skin, cooked)	30 g	2 slices wholemeal bread	7 g
100 g turkey (cooked)	29 g	1 egg (large, hard-boiled)	6 g
100 g tinned tuna (in oil)	27 g	100 g baked beans (salt reduced)	6 g
100 g lamb (lean, cooked)	25 g	2 sardines (tinned in oil)	6 g
100 g fish (bass, cooked)	23 g	28 g almonds/sunflower seeds (handful)	6 g
170 g buckwheat pasta	23 g	100 g cooked brown rice	5 g
100 g kangaroo (cooked)	22 g	28 g cashew nuts/sesame seeds (handful)	5 g
100 g salmon fillet (cooked)	22 g	2 slices rye bread	5 g
100 g smoked salmon	18 g	250 ml soy milk	5 g
100 g lentils (cooked)	9 g	28 g brazil nuts/hazelnuts/pine nuts (handful)	4 g
250 ml sheep milk	15 g	28 g chia seeds	4 g
90 g uncooked oats	11 g	75 g plain, full fat yoghurt	4 g
1 tablespoon hemp seeds	11 g	1 tablespoon spirulina	4 g
250 ml goat milk	9 g	1 cacao nib	4 g
100 g quinoa (cooked)	4 g	1 tablespoon cashew butter/tahini	3 g
100 g tofu	8 g	1 tablespoon almond butter	2 g
250 ml full cream milk	8 g	1 tbsp miso paste	2 g
28 g pumpkin seeds, walnuts (handful)	7 g	8 g Udo's Beyond Greens (1 tablespoon)	2 g
2 egg whites (raw)	7 g	30 ml Udo's 3-6-9 Oil Blend (2 tablespoons)	0.5 g

Vegans and vegetarians need to look at protein content with every meal. Aim to consume 0.8 grams of protein per kilogram of body weight per day.

VEGAN AND VEGETARIAN PROTEIN SOURCES INCLUDE:

- Dairy: yoghurt, sheep or goat's cheese, eggs
- Nuts, seeds, chia seeds, LSA (linseed, sunflower and almond mix)
- Seaweeds: agar agar, kombu, wakame, kelp, nori
- Vegetables: brussels sprouts, parsley, broccoli
- Grains: barley, corn, rye, millet, buckwheat, oats, amaranth, quinoa, wild rice, bulgur, wheat
- Legumes: adzuki beans, dried peas, lentils, chickpeas, kidney beans, black beans, baked beans
- Micro-algae: chlorella, spirulina
- Fermented foods: tamari, sourdough bread, miso, tempeh, tofu (but try to avoid too many soy products).

To ensure that you are eating 'complete' proteins (full of all essential amino acids), eat grains with some kind of bean or seed; for example:

- Millet with adzuki beans
- Rice with beans
- Oats with chia seeds and almonds
- Almonds with brazil nuts and cashew nuts (ABC nut butter – a 'complete' protein)
- Rice or corn with beans
- Brown rice with sunflower seeds
- Corn, buckwheat, quinoa or rye with beans or peas

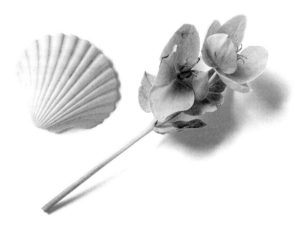

NET DIARY

TIME	PLACE	WITH WHOM	FOOD EATEN AND AMOUNT	FEELINGS BEFORE	FEELINGS AFTER
	At home, on the run, rest, office	Alone, family, friends, work	What you ate, and how much you ate	Hungry, stressed, bored, tired or other	Satisfied, guilty, full, bloated or other
6.00 a.m.					
8.00 a.m.					
10.00 a.m.					
12.00 p.m.					
2.00 p.m.					
4.00 p.m.					
6.00 p.m.					
8.00 p.m.					
10.00 p.m.					
12.00 a.m.					

ENERGY LEVELS: low, med, high

8.00 a.m.

10.00 a.m.

12.00 p.m.

2.00 p.m.

4.00 p.m.

6.00 p.m.

8.00 p.m.

THOUGHTS/FEELINGS:
Happy, sad, overwhelmed, exhausted, irritable, angry, energised?

WATER CONSUMPTION: 750 ml on rising, mid-morning, mid-afternoon, evening

BOWEL MOTIONS: Frequency, any problems

SYMPTOMS: Congestion, constipation, bloating, cramps, headaches, etc.

EXERCISE:

TIME:

TYPE:

INTENSITY:

DURATION:

BIBLIOGRAPHY

Baker, S, *Detoxification and Healing: The Key to Optimal Health*, McGraw-Hill, New York, 2004.

Baroody, T, *Alkalize or Die*, Holographic Health Press, Waynesville, NC, 1991.

Chopra, D, *The Seven Spiritual Laws of Success: A Practical Guide to the Fulfilment of Your Dream*s, Amber-Allen Publishing and New World Library, CA, 1994.

Crook, W & Jones, M, *The Yeast Connection Cookbook*, Professional Books, Tennessee, 1997.

Das, S, *Awakening the Buddha Within: Eight Steps to Enlightenment: Tibetan Wisdom for the Western World*, Broadway Books, New York, 1997.

Diamond, H & M, *Fit for Life Living Health*, Bantam, Great Britain,1992.

Eady, J, *Additive Alert,* Additive Alert, Bayswater WA, 2004.

Erasmus, U, *Fats that Heal, Fats that Kill*, Alive Books, BC, 1993.

Feuerstein, G, *The Shambhala Guide to Yoga*, Shambhala Publications, Inc., Massachusetts, 1996.

French, R, *Natural Health and Vegetarian Life*, 2006.

Gibran, K, *The Prophet*, Penguin, London, 2002.

Hanley, J & Deville, N, *Tired of Being Tired*, Berkley Publishing Group, New York, 2001.

Hidgon, J, *Essential Fatty Acids*, Linus Pauling Institute, Oregon State University, 2005.

Kempton, S, *Meditation for the Love of It*, Sounds True, Louisville, 2011.

Manfield, C, *Tasting India*, Penguin, Melbourne, 2011.

McKeith, G, *You Are What You Eat*, Penguin, Melbourne, 2004.

Murray, M, *Encyclopaedia of Nutritional Supplements*, Prima Publishing, CA, 1996.

Murray, M & Pizzorno, J, *Encyclopaedia of Natural Medicine*, Little Brown & Company, London, 1998.

Noaks, M & Clifton, P, *The CSIRO Total Wellbeing Diet*, Penguin Books, Victoria, 2005.

Osiecki, H, *The Nutrient Bible* (4th ed), Bio Concepts Publishing, Queensland, 2000.

Pitchford, P, *Healing With Whole Foods: Oriental Traditions and Modern Nutrition*, North Atlantic Books, California, 1993.

Pollan, M, *Food Rules: An Eater's Manual*, Penguin Books, Victoria, 2009.

Santillo, H *Intuitive Eating*, Hohm Press, Arizona, 1993.

Shelef, L, 'Antimicrobial effects of spices', *Journal of Food Safety*, pp 29–44.

Snyder, P, 'Antimicrobial effects of spices and herbs', *Hospitality Institute of Technology and Managemen*t, St Paul, Minnesota, 1997.

Statham, B, *The Chemical Maze: Your Guide to Food Additives and Cosmetic Ingredients*, possibilit.com, Victoria, 2002.

Tortora, G & Grabowski, S, *Principles of Anatomy and Physiology*, (9th ed), John Wiley & Sons, Inc, New York, 2000.

Tunsky, G, *The Battle For Health Is Over pH*, Crusador, Orlando, 2004.

Young, R & Redford Young, S, *The pH Miracle*, Warner Books, New York, 2002.

INDEX

ACKNOWLEDGEMENTS

A big thank you to the Penguin team for their hard work in bringing this book to fruition, especially to Julie Gibbs for her knowledge and expertise, my editor Jocelyn Hungerford for her meticulous work, Emily O'Neill for her amazing design and Rob Palmer for his beautiful photography. Also Hanna Marton, for helping to make my raw writing readable.

Heartfelt thanks to my agent Tara Wynne, for accompanying me on this journey, and for your unwavering support. Alexis Elliot, Zoë Foster, Johnny Gannon, Graeme Jolly, Mike Porra and Danielle Ragenard for lending a hand in making this book possible. A special thanks to my friend Antonia Leigh for believing in me. My two best friends, Emma Barnes and Gaby Michaelides – your life-long friendship has made me into the person I am today.

To my clients at The Last Resort, I have learnt so much from you. Thank you for allowing me to accompany you on your journey. To my staff, especially my manager Aimee Suriajaya, thank you for understanding me. Also for your passion and commitment to the work we do. To the naturopaths who have taught me – especially Graeme Bradshaw and Kira Sutherland – thank you for your wisdom and guidance.

To the gorgeous people who didn't think twice about being part of this book – Victoria Alexander, Russ Ayres, Taj Burrow, Maeve Dermody, Alex Dimitriades, Camilla Freeman-Topper, Jessica Gomes, Samantha Harris, Lorraine Wilson, Christine Manfield, Pete Melov, Derek Rielly, David Thompson and Damian Walshe-Howling. A special thanks to the stunning Miranda Kerr for her continued support.

To my family – Daddy, Sam, Abs, Anna, Farrah, Kyra and Ethan – I love you all dearly. My gorgeous in-laws, thank you for making me part of the family. A special thanks to Margaret and David Miller for your love and support. To my gorgeous nieces and nephews, thank you for making me smile. To my goddaughters Bronte Hudson and Daisy Dunn, I am blessed to be a godmother to such divine beings.

To Kalan and Leilani – it is your generosity in your heart and kindness in your nature that guides me. Thank you for your unconditional love.

To my husband and the love of my life, Dan Miller. You are everything to me – my soul-mate, my rock, my best friend, my business partner. Thank you for believing in me, and for holding me and never letting go. Thank you also for building such a divine spa and our special place, Kookie Hill Retreat. I am truly blessed to walk this life with you.

This book is dedicated to my mother, who suffered terribly but never showed it. It was you who taught me about love, humility, strength and compassion.

With love and light,

SAIMAA X

LANTERN

Published by the Penguin Group
Penguin Group (Australia)
707 Collins Street, Melbourne, Victoria 3008, Australia
(a division of Penguin Australia Pty Ltd)
Penguin Group (USA) Inc.
375 Hudson Street, New York, New York 10014, USA
Penguin Group (Canada)
90 Eglinton Avenue East, Suite 700, Toronto, Canada ON M4P 2Y3
(a division of Penguin Canada Books Inc.)
Penguin Books Ltd
80 Strand, London WC2R 0RL England
Penguin Ireland
25 St Stephen's Green, Dublin 2, Ireland
(a division of Penguin Books Ltd)
Penguin Books India Pvt Ltd
11 Community Centre, Panchsheel Park, New Delhi – 110 017, India
Penguin Group (NZ)
67 Apollo Drive, Rosedale, North Shore 0632, New Zealand
(a division of Penguin New Zealand Pty Ltd)
Penguin Books (South Africa) (Pty) Ltd
Rosebank Office Park, Block D, 181 Jan Smuts Avenue, Parktown North,
Johannesburg 2196, South Africa
Penguin (Beijing) Ltd
7F, Tower B, Jiaming Center, 27 East Third Ring Road North,Chaoyang District,
Beijing 100020, China

Penguin Books Ltd, Registered Offices: 80 Strand, London, WC2R 0RL, England

First published by Penguin Group (Australia), 2012

10 9 8 7 6 5 4 3 2

Text copyright © Saimaa Miller 2012
Photography copyright © Rob Palmer 2012

The moral right of the author has been asserted

Cover and text design by Emily O'Neill © Penguin 2012
Styling by Vanessa Austin
Food preparation by Tina Asher
Props provided by Mud Australia, Porters Paints, Dulux and Robert Gordon
Excerpt from *Awakening the Buddha Within: Tibetan Wisdom for the Western World* by Lama Surya Das
copyright © 1997 by Lama Surya Das. Used by permission of Broadway Books, a division of Random House, Inc.
Typeset in Garamond by Post Pre-Press Group, Brisbane, Queensland
Colour reproduction by Splitting Image Colour Studio Pty Ltd, Clayton, Victoria
Printed and bound in China by 1010 Printing International Limited

National Library of Australia
Cataloguing-in-Publication entry:

Miller, Saimaa
Aussie Body Diet & Detox Plan / Saimaa Miller

9780670075911 (pbk)
Includes index.

Diet – Australia
Diet therapy – Australia
Detoxification (Health) – Australia
Nutrition – Australia
Food habits – Australia

613.20994

penguin.com.au/lantern